The Health Collection
provided by
Genesis Health Services
Foundation

Dealing with Doctors, Denial, and Death

Dealing with Doctors, Denial, and Death

A Guide to Living Well with Serious Illness

AROOP MANGALIK, MD

ROWMAN & LITTLEFIELD
Lanham • Boulder • New York • London

Published by Rowman & Littlefield
A wholly owned subsidary of The Rowman & Littlefield Publishing Group, Inc.
4501 Forbes Boulevard, Suite 200, Lanham, Maryland 20706
www.rowman.com

Unit A, Whitacre Mews, 26-34 Stannary Street, London SE11 4AB

British Library Cataloguing in Publication Information Available

Library of Congress Cataloging-in-Publication Data
Names: Mangalik, Aroop, 1935– author.
Title: Dealing with doctors, denial, and death : a guide to living well with serious illness / Aroop Mangalik.
Description: Lanham, Maryland : Rowman & Littlefield, [2017] | Includes bibliographical references and index.
Identifiers: LCCN 2016025054 (print) | LCCN 2016033078 (ebook) | ISBN 9781442272804 (cloth : alk. paper) | ISBN 9781442272811 (electronic)
Subjects: LCSH: Chronically ill—Care. | Chronically ill—Family relationships. | Chronically ill—Treatment. | Physician and patient. | Medical ethics.
Classification: LCC RC108 .M366 2017 (print) | LCC RC108 (ebook) | DDC 616/.044—dc23
LC record available at https://lccn.loc.gov/2016025054

♾™ The paper used in this publication meets the minimum requirements of American National Standard for Information Sciences—Permanence of Paper for Printed Library Materials, ANSI/NISO Z39.48-1992.

Printed in the United States of America

This book is dedicated to John (Jack) H. Saiki,
friend and inspiration

The dimensions of illness extend far beyond the symptoms and physical signs to include the far reaching impact on mind and spirit. We are trained with an emphasis on the biology of disease and its treatment. To the patient and family, the meaning and impact of serious illness is the more significant problem. This "other side" of illness I learned from my patients.

—John H. Saiki, MD, 2011

Contents

Preface

The importance of the problem of pain before one dies is becoming increasingly recognized around the world. With advancing technology and more medical expertise, there is hope for successful treatment of many diseases that were once almost invariably fatal. At the same time, these technologies are causing a prolongation of the process of dying—often painfully.

The word "pain" most often conjures up the agony of a broken bone, a burn or a severe muscle spasm. In this book, however, I will use "pain" to refer to any seriously distressing symptom, including the pressure of a tumor, shortness of breath and even guilt at burdening one's loved ones.

No one wants to suffer needlessly; yet this is happening. The question I ask is "Why do we 'choose' to suffer?" This book gives an analysis of the background and reasons for this paradox. It also provides guidance for patients and their families on how to avoid unnecessary suffering. I often use the second person—"you"—to refer to the seriously ill patient. I do this not because I assume that everyone who reads this book is currently very sick but to put the reader into the frame of mind to think about what he or she would want when faced with a life-threatening illness and, ultimately, death. True, some people die immediately from trauma (being hit by the proverbial bus) or from a sudden event like a heart attack or stroke. But nowadays most Americans die as a result of progressive illness that is partially treatable. This gives them time to make choices about the treatment and care they want—and do not want—at the end of life. The best time to ask yourself what you do, and don't, want is when you are in good health, but whether you are currently healthy or ill, giving consideration to this issue, and discussing it with your doctors and loved ones, will prepare you and your family for you to have a comfortable, peaceful death.

Having worked for 50 years as a hematologist-oncologist, I have interacted with many patients with blood diseases and cancer. In some cases, my patients had good results; in others, the outcome was not so good. Although I tried to minimize the discomfort of my patients, some did die painfully. I have worked in India and in the United States, and during my annual visits to India, I have heard many stories of people who died after prolonged suffering.

After many years of delay, the topic of comfort at death is receiving more attention. Two recent books have drawn attention to this issue. They are insightful and well written, and I cite them often in the chapters that follow. One is by a journalist, Katy Butler (*Knocking on Heaven's Door*), and the other by an Indian-American physician, Atul Gawande (*Being Mortal*). Both authors describe the many problems in the American medical system and some ways to correct them.

Butler's work is about her elderly father's mental deterioration and both of her parents' frailty. She describes how they suffered for many years and were not able to die in peace. Gawande's book also describes his father's illness and suffering in the later years of life. In addition, Gawande looks at the problems that arise with aging and how to cope with them.

The present book goes further into the analysis of the role of the medical establishment (defined broadly) and of doctors in contributing to physical and emotional pain of people as they age, get sick and approach death. In the pages that follow, you will learn about the psychology, education and training of physicians, along with the professional and cultural environment in which they work. These often lead to their subjecting patients to tests and procedures that have little, if any, chance of benefiting their patients. This book also offers suggestion of what you, as a patient, can do to avoid this over-treatment.

This book is written primarily for people who are interested in taking charge of their lives and their deaths. Whether you are currently ill or in the best of health, it should help you in making your own choices about a crucial issue and making sure your wishes are carried out.

Introduction

Our mother was very sick. My older sister was 10 years old. She went to visit Amma in the hospital but was not allowed to go into the room. She was then sent to boarding school. When she came back for the holidays, she asked, "Where is Amma?" Of course, Amma had died, but no one had told Meera about it.

Different cultures, different families and different individuals respond to death in their own ways. Understanding or even having some knowledge about the reactions to death and its inevitability is helpful. When we face the end directly, that understanding facilitates the process of dealing with the anguish, regrets and "what ifs" of death.

As outsiders, we must be sensitive to other peoples' reactions to death, which is too personal for us to judge. Many social and circumstantial factors come into play. The following two anecdotes illustrate why we should not judge other cultures and the circumstances that lead to the reactions or practices they have.

A particularly insensitive remark by General William Westmoreland, who was the man most responsible for implementing the escalation of the Vietnam War in the mid-1960s, was quoted in his obituary in the *New York Times*. Referring to the Vietnamese, Westmoreland said, "The Oriental doesn't put the same price on life as the Westerner. Life is plentiful, life is cheap in the Orient."[1] This statement is appalling and reflects the speaker's lack of cultural awareness.

Another example involves the practices of one tribe in Sub-Saharan Africa. Knowing that I was interested in cultural attitudes about the end of life, a friend told me that this tribe often needed to migrate in search of water. On one of these migrations, the chief was mauled by a lion. He was not likely to recover. Even though he was their leader, the tribe decided to leave him to die because carrying him would jeopardize the rest of the group. This was their reality, and it was acceptable to them.

An often-repeated statement is that death is a part of life and will happen to all living things—in a few minutes for bacteria, in a few years or decades for mammals and in a few thousand years for the mighty redwoods. Yet we often lead our lives as if death will not happen to us. In the Mahabharata, one of the great Indian epics, a young man asks a wise person, "What is the most wondrous thing on earth?" The sage replied, "Every day people die, but those who are living keep on believing that they are immortal. What can be more wondrous than that?"[2]

It is *this* phenomenon of personal denial that I would like to explore. The role of society, religion and ourselves in this process is intriguing and not clearly understood. Philosophers, religious leaders, psychologists and scholars have tried to deal with it. Many books have been written, seminars held and issues constantly debated, sometimes contentiously. Archeologists and anthropologists have ascribed many of the findings from excavations and traditional ceremonies to those cultures' attempts to deal with death. From around the world and from finds 15,000 years old to recent ones, one can see altars, monoliths and burial sites suggesting human concerns about death.

What I have read about the topic has been somewhat useful. However, many of the texts have been difficult to understand because they were written for specialists in the fields of philosophy, religion and ethics. There are also "handbooks" compiled by palliative care and hospice personnel. Palliative-care physicians are trained in methods for controlling the symptoms that result from serious illness. People who work in hospice help people die in peace and comfort. They get involved in the patient's care when it has been decided that there should be no further attempt to treat the underlying disease, and their focus is on comfort for the patient and the family until death occurs. These books have helped a lot, but they do not include an analysis of the perceptions of death and do not look into the "most wondrous thing"—denial of mortality. In this book I deal with the practical issues surrounding life's end, with the goal of helping people understand what they can do to reduce the burdens of aging, illness and death. This begins with thinking and talking about what may happen. I explain the systemic pressures that can lead to difficulties. This book also provides usable information to those who want to have a good life, right up to its end, and a good death.

I have been involved with patients with cancer for nearly 50 years and for 20 of those years have been advocating to reduce treatments that are painful and have no chance of helping the patient. I have learned a lot about suffering and death. I have learned about denial and acceptance. I have seen comfortable deaths with family and friends around the dying person, and I have seen people suffer before they die.

This book is written mainly for the non-medical public—those who have no formal training in the field. However, "non-medical" may be a misnomer. With our aging population and the use of more medical technologies, there is hardly anyone who has not become acquainted with the treatments for serious illness or who has not experienced death in her family or among his circle of friends. I believe a wide audience will find my analysis useful, since it is presented without jargon or technical language, with clear statements and without ambiguity—a style that I appreciate when things outside my own field are explained to me.

Medical professionals may also find my approach useful. In my five decades as a physician, I have had many experiences in two cultures. I did my medical training in India and the United States and have worked as a doctor in both countries, giving me a somewhat different perspective that American medical professionals may find interesting. I am a part of both cultures but not fully immersed in either. My view on this can be expressed by a saying in Hindi (my mother tongue), which translates roughly: "I am of the world, but am not enamored of the world. I am in the marketplace, but am not a buyer." This attitude of mine may be refreshing to some but annoying to others. My approach toward painful treatments with low chance of benefit is different from that of many in the United States. I am also more accepting of the inevitability of death than most Americans. In addition to working as an oncologist, I have studied and taught medical ethics. This has given me a broader perspective about medicine.

From my experiences with patients, families and colleagues and from my readings, I have, at the suggestion of a friend, put together some thoughts, some ideas and a perspective on death that I hope may be helpful. Another book about death is needed, I think, to come to grips with a reality we often try to forget. To protect the privacy of patients and colleagues, I have often changed names and other identifying features. In the cases of the medical students and the young physicians whom I have trained and who generously shared their illustrative experiences, I have used their own words with their permission and have identified them by name.

As I write this book, a thought keeps coming to me: Am I undermining the trust that patients and people at large have in doctors? Trust is essential in person-to-person interactions. Seller and buyer, negotiators and family should trust each other if their interaction is to be positive.

Similarly, mutual trust between patients and doctors is critical for the appropriate delivery of treatments and for health care in general. Yes, throughout this book I have written about the health-care system and the people in it—medical and non-medical—and have pointed out problems and misdeeds. My aim in this is to make patients and families aware of certain realities and how these could affect them; it is not to break trust or confidence. The health-care *system* in the United States has many problems, some of which I address. Having worked in the system for many years, I have met and collaborated with a large number of health-care professionals. I have encountered very few whom I did not trust or like. But there have been a few exceptions, and I have written about some of their actions that I felt were wrong. The system has problems, and I have brought these to the reader's attention. I have made some general suggestions for improving the system, but a detailed discussion of that is out of the scope of this book and beyond my expertise.

I hope that what I have written will provide insight into how people in general, patients and families and also doctors react to and deal with serious illnesses and death, and I have expanded on some of these points to guide those facing these difficult situations. This book looks at the problem from the perspectives of both the medical provider and the patient. My primary aim is to help you, as a patient, understand your situation and your rights.

This book does not tell you or your doctors what should and should not be done, but it attempts to help you make appropriate and informed decisions. After all, it is your life, your illness and your death.

Dealing with the Inevitability of Death

Death. It is a fact of life. How we deal with it and why we do what we do about it is a bigger and more relevant topic.

The inevitability of death also brings into focus the finality of death. Yes, death is the final event in the cycle of life, and that makes it hard to face. Every person, healthy or sick, young or old, religious or nonbeliever, educated or not, faces death in his or her own way. People and groups also vary in the way they deal with death. I begin with three examples from my own family.

My mother died in 1941 in her thirties, my father died in 1962 at the age of 61, and my father-in-law died in 2006 at the age of 89. Each death was different.

When my mother died, I was only five years old. In the era before antibiotics were widely available, she developed an acute gallbladder infection complicated by infection of the blood (septicemia). I remember her being sick at home, transported back and forth to the hospital, and then not returning home. As I mentioned briefly in the introduction, my sister Meera, the oldest, was ten. She went to the hospital to see Amma but was not allowed to go into the room. She was sent away to a boarding school. When she came back for the holidays, she asked, "Where is Amma?" Of course, Amma had died, but no one had told Meera about it. No one in the family had told my brother and me, either. We were sent to stay with an uncle who lived in town and learned of our mother's death from our schoolmates. That was the way my family handled death.

We did not grieve for Amma, and we did not talk about her. Life went on without her as if everything were normal. I cannot explain why my family tried to cover up my mother's death; perhaps it was due to my physician father's training with British doctors, many from the Royal Indian Army Medical Corps. They may have inculcated in him the idea of being stoic and not yielding to one's emotions. At any rate, that was what happened.

I was not affected at a conscious level at the time, but over the years, it has become clear that some of my personality traits can be traced to those early years. The memory of the way my mother's death was handled did have an impact on my attitude toward death when I became a health-care provider. I have been an advocate for open communication about illness and death for over 25 years.

Papa's death at the age of 61 was sad, and, in retrospect, I can see how it, too, has affected my attitude toward communication and honesty in the face of serious illness. This includes acceptance of death when medical reality clearly shows that control of the disease is not feasible and death is likely in the near future. The events and the actions taken by all those involved and affected by his illness did not include discussions, honest appraisal or the acceptance of a death that was clearly imminent. I will describe the events, the way the illness proceeded, and the consequences of avoiding the reality. This occurred more than 50 years ago. Attitudes were different then; there were many social factors influencing the thinking and actions of the doctors and the family. The point is not to judge but to try to understand what happened then and prevent the same from happening to others in the future.

My father was in excellent health all his life, active mentally and physically. He retired at age 60, as was mandatory in the Indian system. He was a professor of pathology at Lucknow, one of the oldest medical colleges in India. To keep his mind occupied and transmit his knowledge and experience to others, he accepted an assignment with the World Health Organization. He went to Burma (now Myanmar) to teach at a medical college that needed help. He worked there for about a year and returned home for the summer break. At this point, my sister Meera and I were both in Delhi. I was in my residency training at the fairly new but prestigious All India Institute of Medical Sciences (AIIMS). My sister and her young family were at an air force base where her husband, a pilot, was posted.

Shortly after returning home, Papa started complaining of episodes of shortness of breath. At first, these happened every few days; then they started occurring daily. Through his own contacts and because of my being at the AIIMS, we consulted the head of cardiology there. There was no abnormality found on examination or through the tests that were done. However, the episodes of shortness of breath continued. Papa returned to Lucknow, our hometown. There, too, he had very knowledgeable and competent physicians. Again, the cause of the symptoms could not be found. He continued to receive treatments that partially relieved them, but overall his condition kept getting worse. It was determined that the problem was in his heart, but it was not clear what kind of defect he had. Because his condition was deteriorating, he was moved to the AIIMS in Delhi so that he could be under the care of the best available cardiologist and because I was working in that hospital. He was evaluated by other doctors, but his disease remained undiagnosed. Treatments for his failing heart were continued and modified according to the need of the day, but the overall situation and his symptoms of shortness of breath and fluid build-up continued. It was clear that he was dying, but no one talked about it. Was it denial or poor communication? I cannot say.

This is where the issues of communication and facing the truth come in. Of course, this is in retrospect, after I have thought about the situation many times over the years. On the one hand, as I reflected on what happened before my father's death, I became conscious of what should have been done. On the other, as I became aware of the need for communication and honesty, I became more and more aware of what we missed out on. We did not say good-byes; we never said, "I love you, I will miss you"; and we never had closure.

Lamenting itself is not of much value, but if we learn from the past, we can improve the situation for the future. We should not forget that all this happened in the early 1960s. At that time, discussion of the medical situation with patient or family was not the norm. If the prognosis was bad, there was even less communication, as if talking about the likely dire outcome would bring it about. It seems that no one thought how devastating the effect of death would be on the family if they did not realize how grave the situation was.

Simple knowledge of medicine will lead to the conclusion that if a patient has heart failure whose cause cannot be identified and the best available treatments are not producing any benefit and the patient's condition is getting worse, he will die in the near future. During my training, I had had other patients with heart failure who did die in the hospital. We did not talk about their impending deaths. We did not counsel the patient or the family.

The only difference was that with those patients, we knew the cause of the heart failure.

So life and Papa's illness coasted along. It was now over three months that he had been in the hospital just sitting in bed with oxygen, not able to interact much, all of us sad, even glum. Some out-of-town family came to visit. We talked pleasantries, but no one asked, "Now what?"

One morning, my father suddenly collapsed; his blood pressure dropped to very low levels. His doctors gave him fluids by vein, and his blood pressure came up. He actually had less shortness of breath than he had had for several months, and he was more interactive. We did not accept that he had had a further setback. We were happy that he felt better for a few hours. Out-of-town family members were called and asked to come to Delhi. Again, no further discussion! Papa, in fact, asked, "Is my condition worse?" The response was "No, no. Everything is fine." This would have been a good time to talk openly, but that did not happen.

When Papa saw the family members who came from out of town, he asked, "Why are you here?" and the response was "I just happened to have work in Delhi!" Again, no one acknowledged that he was about to die.

We went along as before. Papa's appetite was somewhat better, and his breathing was easier, so we just celebrated that, imagining, maybe believing, that this was the beginning of his recovery.

The doctors came to see Papa more frequently throughout the day. I spent the whole day in his room—but there was no discussion of "What now?" Then, late that night, Papa's heart stopped. Attempts were made to revive him, but he was declared dead after his doctors finally accepted the situation. Why had there been attempts at cardio-pulmonary resuscitation (CPR) in someone whose heart function had been deteriorating for several months? Because that was the way we did things. Why no communication? Why no discussion of what would happen? That was the way things were done in those days. Have we improved half a century later? Are we doing a better job?

The short answer is "No." Many doctors do not initiate the discussion about a bad medical situation, and many families do not want to face the reality. But now, at last, we are starting to see a trend toward honesty, openness and acceptance.

I have learned the importance of honesty and openness. I have talked about this to my family, friends, students and colleagues. I see evidence of more and better communication in my medical students. Also, nationally the idea of facing life-threatening illness openly is being accepted more and more.

But we have a long way to go.

The third death of a family member was recent. My father-in-law was nearly 90 and had been active and interactive with his family until a few months before his final illness. He developed some respiratory problems and took simple measures to control them. He found they were not helping. He met with the family and at a certain point said, "I am tired," lay down and died peacefully after a productive life and saying his goodbyes. The family was together; they celebrated his life. This was an example of a good death. He died without pain, without harsh treatments and with his family around him.

At one level, we all know that death is a natural process. It is a part of life. We see it; we read about it; we even talk about it. Children see pets die; the TV news is full of deaths from car wrecks, war, terrorism and natural disasters. But then we draw a line somewhere in our hearts, our minds and our thinking. "Out of sight, out of mind" is the saying that applies to most of us. Yes, death will happen, but why worry about it now? "Denial" is one word sometimes used to describe this phenomenon. I think "denial" applies more accurately to situations where the process is already happening; we are aware of it but don't act or even react to it. If a child shows signs of using drugs or alcohol, one unfortunately common response is that his parents, despite the signs, don't see, or choose not to see, the addiction—they are in denial. If a loved one whose disease is progressing and whose death is near has what the family and others around her call "hope," that is another example of denial. If medical professionals do not discuss the situation honestly with their patients, is that denial?

Before driving off on a long trip, we check different parts of the car, including the paperwork—license, registration and insurance. The chances of something bad happening are small, but we do check—maybe because the documents are in front of us. On the other hand, the certainty of our dying is obvious; only the timing is uncertain. The consequences of not having our personal (death) papers in order are much greater than those of an expired car registration. To use another example, many people are careful in planning for their retirement but do not think of planning for how they would like to die.

Not thinking about or not dealing with a serious situation only increases the harm that will be caused later. Not facing the reality of a serious illness and its consequences will most likely lead to hasty decisions that may not be in the patient's or family's best interest. This phenomenon of denial occurs in many situations and is quite common. We need to overcome this natural tendency so as to avoid problems for ourselves and those around us at a later time. Denial of death occurs, understandably, because death is not easy to think about. But denial causes many difficulties. Understanding why we do not face the problem helps. We do not like to think of death because society does not deal with it. We do what most people around us do. Yet people at some level actually *are* thinking about death. If the topic is brought up, then people will talk about it. Many patients have told me that they will fight and beat their cancer. But when I explain that the cancer in their case is not treatable and will lead to their death, they say, "Yes, I knew that, but I didn't want to think about it." Our mental makeup and our previous experiences or "beliefs" all play a role in the way we deal with bad news and death. It is not a matter of "good" and "bad"; it is a natural and common phenomenon. This point should be helpful in understanding this natural barrier to recognizing and thinking about a dire situation.

Denial of death is a defense mechanism that is common, maybe normal. It allows us, in some way, at least temporarily, to feel that we can avoid the unavoidable. Some have called denial a form of self-delusion. Death is hard on the dying, and death is distressing to those who are still living. But it needs to be faced to avoid unnecessary pain. We often forget that death comes to all of us—including our loved ones and ourselves.

Another reason we do not think of death as "real" is that in our society, death has been sanitized. When a person dies, professionals take the responsibility of preparing the body for the funeral and subsequent cremation or burial. In the funeral home, many times the mourners do not see the dead person. Even when there is an open casket, the body has been transformed with makeup to look like he or she "is only sleeping." This is very different from what occurred in America even a hundred years ago, and it also is different from what occurs today in most of the world.

I am often asked why I take an interest in a sad topic like death. My response is that by thinking and talking about death early on, one can avoid sadness later, and thus it is a happy topic and not a sad one.

There is also the phenomenon of denial by medical providers. Doctors are human beings, and like all of us they have problems facing death.

Some providers deny the reality that a disease is too advanced to be treated. They want to try some treatment or another, despite poor odds. Those who deny the reality of the medical condition deprive their patients of comfort before they die.

There is a parable about Buddha, who lived six centuries before Christ.[1] A wealthy woman's only child, a year-old boy, died, and she was distraught. She pleaded with Buddha to bring her baby back to life. Buddha said he could do that, but only if she brought him four or five mustard seeds from a house where no one had died. Obviously, the woman failed in her quest. In that time and place, people lived in the same house, or at least the same village, their entire lives.

"I have asked you to do the impossible," Buddha admitted. "Every mortal is marked by death. No one can escape it. That is why you could not find a death-free home. This is my lesson to you: Death is universal. We all have to die."

Once the grieving mother accepted the reality of death, she felt some consolation because she realized that it happens to everyone.

In more recent times, psychiatrist Elisabeth Kübler-Ross observed how people deal with bad news, especially life-threatening illness and death.[2] She summarized that we commonly go through certain reactions, often in the order of anger, denial, bargaining, depression and acceptance. The sequence is not fixed, and some people do not go through all these stages. But we all go through many responses to a bad situation. It is normal, human behavior. The point is that when we realize that we have a serious situation on our hands and ultimately accept it, this makes it easier to deal with the reality. However, certain common emotional responses can come into play that prevent us from understanding and accepting.

When I was working in India, I had an experience that still, after 45 years, makes me sad. A man from a poor family had only one son. The father had sacrificed everything for the son's education. The son got a master's degree and was about to start a promising career. Just at that time, he developed acute leukemia, a disease for which there are reasonable treatments currently, but even now only one-third are cured. In those days, people died of the disease in six months to a year. Unfortunately, this young man died. I had been talking to the father on a regular basis and had kept him informed of the serious nature of the illness and the failure of the treatments we had tried. Despite this, several hours after the young man died, the father came to me and said, "He is just sleeping, isn't he? He will be all right." There was no way to console the poor father. All I could do was to sit with him for as long as I could.

These are some questions I would like to explore in the pages that follow. Why do we not prepare for our death? Why we do not talk to our friends and family about death? Why do we cling onto the slimmest of hopes when all signs tell us that death is near and it will happen soon? Why are we willing to endure pain before death?

In recent years there has been more, but not enough, willingness to talk and think about death. Bioethicist Daniel Callahan has educated us about the need for society to change its attitude toward death and to look at transforming the goals of medicine from just treating disease to making life better.[3] Since surgeon Sherwin B. Nuland's bestselling book *How We Die* in 1993, more people consider talking about death acceptable.[4]

Over the years, the patients I have cared for and worked with have had a variety of responses to impending death. However, in most cases, when the medical providers were honest and discussed the issue openly with empathy, the patients accepted the reality. When facing death, the patient and the family may avoid discussing the topic on their own, but deep inside they do understand the situation. When the physician initiates the discussion, they will listen. It gives them "permission" to talk about it. Initiating such a discussion is not easy, even for the experienced and sympathetic provider. But it helps to *ask* the patient and the loved ones about their expectations. It helps further to ask them to separate their hopes from their expectations. Providing medical specifics, filling in details about the disease in general and the way the illness has progressed, further help by providing the patient and family members with greater understanding. A discussion of options and possible courses of action needs to be part of the overall approach to the patient's disease. Are more or different treatments available? What are the pros and cons of the possible treatments?

If death is likely in the near future, it is critical that medical providers explain how it will happen. Most important, it must be made clear that the patient can be kept comfortable up to the time of death. They need to ask where the patient would like to die—at home, in the hospital or in some other facility. The patient can be urged to think of death as a step in the cycle of life and the illness. The approach described is by no means easy for the patient or for those around him. There are many nuances and steps; the discussion takes time and needs to be held with freedom for all concerned to think about the implications of what was discussed. It may take more than one session to come to an understanding and consensus.

What is important is to consider the alternative—if an honest discussion is not held, if the patient has false hopes the situation will be worse. Even after clear and honest discussions, patients may want to continue treatments because of false hope, as chapter 2, "Communication, Hope and Honesty," explains further. The reasons for maintaining false hope are complex and interrelated, both for the patient and for the provider. And false hope often leads to spending precious final days or weeks undergoing painful, futile treatments, instead of setting out on a path to comfort and peace.

2

Communication, Hope and Honesty

Communication is a major component of interaction between living beings. We know it occurs in animals small and large. The degree and nature of this form of interaction seems to be more complex in the species that have evolved more recently. Primates, especially human beings, have many methods of communication.

Communication between humans has multiple facets. It has verbal, visual and body language components. It is not enough just to use the correct words and give facts and figures. The "whole story" should be discussed. Further, communication should be a two-way process; all people involved should be participating for it to be meaningful. We need to listen and to talk. If we make eye contact, it makes the communication more effective. If people show signs of being impatient, communication can be disrupted.

In the medical context, this is especially important. Doctors need to provide information to the patient and family in full detail in a language that is clear and free of technical jargon. Patients for their part must ask questions, get clarifications and feel that they are a part of the process of decision-making and planning. My evolution as a communicator will provide a perspective on communication.

I went to medical school in India in the mid-1950s. Our patients were mostly poor, and many had no formal education. They often had serious illnesses and came to the hospital because they were quite sick. They underwent considerable hardships to get to the hospital. By nature of the social structure, we, as medical students and doctors, were from the middle class or better. This is not the time or place to comment on or be judgmental about India's social structure; that was the reality.

Our communication with patients and their families was mostly in the form of information and instruction. We would tell them that they had a problem with their heart or liver, undertake the treatment in the hospital and give instructions on what to do after they left the hospital and returned to their villages. Many of the illnesses had no long-term solutions, and that was communicated to the patients. There were a few patients who had treatable, indeed curable, conditions like anemia from malnutrition, which we could remedy successfully. That was of course gratifying to the patients and to us.

During my residency training in the United States, there was more attention paid to communication, and some discussions with patients of prognoses and certain details of treatments were undertaken. It was during my specialized training in hematology (blood diseases) that I learned about discussing and explaining to the patient the nature of the illness, the treatments available, the relative efficacy of the treatments and the likely outcome. In those days, there was no treatment available for many of the diseases from which our patients suffered. Maxwell Wintrobe, my mentor (I will refer to him again in chapter 8), was a strong proponent of involving patients in the overall management of their illnesses. From him I learned about open communication, a practice that I have continued and improved upon.

After finishing my training, I returned to India and continued to treat patients with blood diseases and also to teach medical students and resident physicians. I had to modify some of my methods of communication because of the social circumstances, mainly related to the lack of education in many of the patients. Also, I had families who wanted to "protect" patients from bad news. I learned to convince them that the patient needed to be a part of the discussions and decision-making. The families realized that everyone was better off when the discussion was open and frank. Despite this, in retrospect, I can see that I was not always as clear and open then as I am now—a position I strongly advocate.

On returning to the United States to continue my career, I became increasingly aware of the treatments that were being given to patients just because they were available and not because they were expected to help those individuals.

In the 1970s and 1980s, there was a lot of hope that medical science would make breakthroughs, and we were all expected to and did have that hope. A lot of research was being conducted. By signing the National Cancer Act on December 23, 1971, President Richard Nixon had declared "War on Cancer,"[1] and we, myself included, felt we must do "everything" to try to help control the diseases we were dealing with. I found myself accepting many of the advances that were helping patients. At the same time I felt uneasy about the blanket acceptance by many of my colleagues of the idea that more was better. My solution was to talk to my colleagues in academic settings about the idea that more treatment was not necessarily better. I tried to present a more thoughtful approach toward marginal or long-shot treatments. At the same time, I went against the norm when talking to my patients. I did tell them about a particular available new treatment but explained and emphasized that the treatment was not proven and that the chances of benefit for them were small. Once I felt that they understood the good and the bad of the treatment, I let them make the choice. I also gave them the option of talking to another physician before making a final decision.

I did find myself at odds with some of my colleagues but felt comfortable because I helped the patients make informed decisions.

I have made open communication a part of my teaching of medical students and trainees at different levels of their careers. Nationally and in my institution, I have noticed a change. More and more young doctors are accepting the need for and advantages of honesty and openness and that comfort before death is in itself a good goal.

Let us examine each of these points in more detail.

Ideally, doctors should give the patient information about the disease, the expected course of events, what treatments are available and how likely they are to help. Obviously, the details will vary depending on the patient and the disease, but it is the responsibility and obligation of medical providers to give all relevant information to the patient. Further, they should give the patient a chance to seek clarification and ask questions. In the end, the patient should be fully informed and thus able to make an informed decision about what treatment he or she would agree to follow. In reality, this does not always happen. Some doctors communicate clearly, but many do not. Some encourage patients to ask questions; others do not. Some use simple non-technical language; others use technical terms without realizing that medical terms are not a part of the average person's vocabulary. Terms like "cardiac" for heart, "renal" for kidney or "pulmonary" for lungs may not be familiar to non-medical people—doctors forget that. Effort is now being made during the training of young doctors to educate them about the need to use clear, non-technical language.[2]

There have been some interesting and difficult-to-understand responses from some in the medical community and the "right to life" organizations. In 2009 and 2010, California and New York passed legislation to require physicians to explain to patients and families the prognosis and the options available to them. Both laws were designed to ensure that patients were given all the information they requested or *needed* if they had a terminal illness. Note, this was a requirement to provide information, after which the patients would be free to make their own decisions and choose their options.

The California statute was opposed by right to life organizations and some medical professional groups. They claimed it was an "intrusion on the doctor-patient relationship." The New York statute was opposed by some physicians who said this would "generate cynicism at the times when critically ill patients and their families are most in need of honesty, kindness and engagement."[3]

I have read these statements many times and cannot understand how open communication can interfere with the doctor-patient relationship or cause cynicism. My guess is that these people just wanted the patient to have only so-called "positive" information, which is unfair to all concerned.

In the case of a man with a severe head injury, where it was clear there was no chance of recovery, one doctor made a statement that confused the family and made their decision to stop active treatment harder.[4] After saying there was no hope for recovery, he added, "Who knows? Anything can happen." This just made the situation more difficult for the family. Although the statement was nominally true, it only produced confusion by giving the patient's family members false hope.

When providers do talk to patients, there are limitations, making the conversation incomplete or not fully clear. In her *Arizona Law Review* article "Denying Death," University of Utah professor of law and medical ethics Teneille Brown gives several illuminating examples.[5] Some doctors think that if the patient has an advance directive, that is enough. Advance directives are good but really are just the point at which to start the discussion about end-of-life choices. There are many specifics that need to be talked about. Doctors should not wait for the patient and family to initiate the conversation—the doctors should do so. Furthermore, follow-up is very helpful. Another problem is that the time doctors devote to conversations about end-of-life issues has not been properly reimbursed, although this is changing. Medicare now pays physicians $86 for a half-hour discussion of what a patient does and does not want done in case of serious illness.[6]

When doctors do give honest information, they often combine it with some optimistic content. The optimism may not be realistic, but patients tend to focus on those reassuring remarks. For seriously ill, dying patients, the optimism that is important to convey is the assurance that they can be kept comfortable and will not be abandoned. The physician can say "I will fight for you," rather than "We will fight this cancer."

Sometimes, doctors give mixed messages; they combine the good and the bad news. What this leads to is that patients remember only the good news, which may relate to only a small part of the real problem. Thus decisions get made based on false premises.[7]

If patients are not fully informed, they obviously cannot participate in decision-making for their care or treatment. They do not make arrangements to get their financial and other affairs in order. They do not call their loved ones who live far away and ask them for a final visit. Worst of all, patients are unable to make decisions that fit into their goals and values.

On the other side, patients often do not ask for clarification about the information they do not understand. The reasons for this are many. One problem is that many doctors do not support the idea of patients asking questions. Some are haughty and consider themselves to be superior and thus intimidate their patients. If as a patient or family member you encounter this, it can be helpful to ask one of the doctor's co-workers to help you. Often a nurse is able to explain the disease and treatment in clear terms. Take advantage of that. A study from the University of Queensland found that patients often turned to nurses for emotional support.[8] Alex Broom, an Australian sociologist specializing in health and illness, explained, "A major problem is that some doctors avoid difficult conversations, even continuing patients on active treatments, while others were rushed or blunt, leaving the nurse to explain the situation and provide emotional support to the patients and their families."[9]

Another unfortunate reality is that some patients become fearful and childlike when they are sick. This has been described by oncologist Jerome Groopman in his book *Your Medical Mind*.[10] He cites the case of a professor of English who was articulate and forceful in his professional life. However, when faced with an encounter with his surgeon, he said, "Each time I got with the surgeon, it was as if my mind went out the window. I was like a frightened child in front of him and couldn't think at all." My father-in-law, whom I mentioned earlier, was well versed in history and economics. He had meaningful discussions on a variety of topics with different people. However, when he returned from a visit to his doctor, he could not describe what the doctor had said. He could only say, "The doctor did these tests and gave me these pills."

Thus, when doctors do not communicate properly and patients accept that, the patients make uninformed decisions. Further, this lack of communication may contribute to the growing phenomenon of unnecessary, even unwanted, treatments. Let us look at how and why doctors fail to communicate adequately information regarding the disease, the expected outcomes and the kinds of treatments available.

Patients will often go for a treatment based on the best possible scenario. However, the best possible scenario may just be improvement of heart function by "x" percent for two months, without making the patient feel better. In deciding whether to accept or reject a given treatment, you as the patient must at least know what the best possible outcome is. A doctor's just saying that there is a new treatment that may work is unfair, in fact deceptive. The best possible scenario may or may not be good enough for you. Further, how often does the "best" occur? If only one in 20 patients has improvement, you may not consider the odds acceptable. Also, you need to know what "improvement" really means and whether, in particular, "improvement" means that you will feel better.

Many medical providers are honest; they talk to their patients and explain the situation to them. They describe what ails the patient and why (assuming they can determine that). They say what they know, and they suggest what can make the patient better or at least how they can make the patient *feel* better. Many doctor-patient encounters go well to the satisfaction of both parties, but not all do.

When dealing with serious illness, life-changing or life-threatening, the problem is magnified, and both parties need to adjust. The discussion has to be modified and adapted to the specific circumstance. When it comes to complicated issues and when bad news needs to be delivered, the situation becomes even more difficult. The discussion of the nature of the problem will be different if, for example, an otherwise healthy patient has a hernia or if he has cancer of the pancreas and a major surgery to remove that diseased organ is being considered.

Our system of medical education is heavily focused on providing the facts about anatomy, physiology, genetics, biochemistry, pathology and pharmacology, to name just a few. Our medical students (and doctors) are knowledgeable in these and other matters of science and medicine. Until recently, very little effort and time was spent on teaching students and young doctors about how patients feel, how to understand them or how to communicate with them. As a result, many doctors who are good at diagnosis and treatment do not do a good job of understanding their patients and also are not able to explain themselves to their patients.

Teneille Brown further states, "Our culture generally denies death, but seems to be even more reluctant to acknowledge its presence in the face of terminal cancer. For cultural, legal and *financial* reasons, cancer patients receive overly aggressive care [treatment] at the EOL [end of life]."[11]

She goes on to say, "[T]his aggressive care is often provided under false pretenses, as the patients assume the treatments can cure their cancer, even though the providers hold out no such hope for a cure."[12]

This is changing. More time and effort is being made across the country to teach communication methods to our young students and trainees. Unfortunately, there are many doctors who have not had the benefit of this important field of training. They continue to struggle with themselves about how to communicate effectively. They speak in a way that is difficult for the patient to understand. They use technical terms rather than everyday language. They are so used to medical terminology that they fail to realize that not everybody has exposure to words that they utilize commonly with their colleagues. They also make statements that are not clear or definitive. They use double negatives. "This drug is not so good but not using it may not be helpful." On the other hand, they may over-simplify. They may tell the patient that this treatment will give you three more months of life. The reality of course is that no one knows how long a person is going to live. The fact is that with this particular treatment *on average* patients have lived three months longer than with previous treatments. This limited communication is one of the reasons why doctors give treatments that may have an effect on the disease but do not help the patients. This is because patients receive false hope and agree to take treatments that may not benefit them.

Hope is a natural feeling when one is faced with a serious illness. Good communication needs to be honest, but it can still provide hope. The doctor needs to explain that even if the disease cannot be controlled, there is *hope* because there are ways to keep the patient comfortable. If patients are assured that they will not be abandoned, this can be healing even if not curing. Most patients like to continue to be supported by their own doctors. It means a lot to them to know that their doctor will be available if they need her.

Such communication and assurance avoids the use of futile treatments— treatments that do not control the disease and do not make the patient feel better. The "combat mentality" that many of us physicians have is not helpful. Rather than focusing on fighting and winning, we need to look at how we can make the best of a bad situation.

Time and empathy are other facets of communication that are helpful to patients who are facing difficult situations and have to make difficult decisions. They need time, and they need to be listened to empathically. Silence is considered by some experts to be a method of communication. When patients are told that they have a damaged liver or a failing heart, such information is disconcerting. Patients need time to process what the doctor has said, to think of what it could mean. They need the opportunity to formulate the questions they want to ask.

During a session on "meaningful encounters," I have had many students describe how just listening or even just "being there" was helpful to the patients and meaningful to the students themselves. In these sessions, students describe stories of patients that left a significant impression on them.

Here are some excerpts from their essays.

a. Sarah Cordova's experience with a 56-year-old man with a rapidly progressive, untreatable cancer

I was at my limit as a medical student. So suddenly without thinking I asked if I could give them a hug. It seemed like instantly they all smiled and jumped to hug me. The wife told me thank you and said that I touched their lives and they will never forget me. It was at that moment that I felt the most fulfillment and happiness I have felt since starting med school. I had not done anything more than show I cared, but that was all that they needed in that moment. It made me realize that being a doctor is so much more than medical knowledge.

b. Page Pomo's experience with a woman facing disability and dependence on others

Sometimes I would hardly talk, and instead just sit and listen to her express her concerns and anxieties about her condition or about how much she missed her family in El Paso. She would tell me about how she enjoyed painting and jewelry-making before this disease took its toll on her body. Now she struggles to lift her arms to feed herself, and was confined to a bed 24 hours a day. Yet, patient's like Ms. M, with her daily gratitude and courageous spirit, reminded me why I chose medicine as my career. Not so I could sit behind a computer all day, but so I could interact with patients in a meaningful and lasting way. I may not succeed in curing every patient, but sometimes the best "cure" is offering genuine concern—a listening ear, a warm smile—and simply supporting a patient through a difficult season of life.

c. Kyle Leggott's description of a man with bleeding from his stomach

I followed a patient specifically because I thought he would be someone who could benefit from therapeutic listening. Over the next few days, there was a noticeable change in the patient; the more he was able to tell his story the more upbeat and interactive he was. By the end, we had not done much for physical symptom control, but we had made him feel significantly better just by listening and reassuring him that we were there to help him.

Doctors often give the information about diagnosis and recommended treatment and describe what may happen. Then, without a pause, they say, "Any questions?" They wait a few moments and leave the room. This is a bit of an exaggeration, but a common enough occurrence to leave many a patient bewildered. Silence to allow patients to gather their thoughts is very important. This needs to be followed by another step—the opportunity to express their thoughts, their fears and their understanding of the news given to them by the doctor. Just asking the patient "Any questions?" is not enough. A doctor needs to make the patient comfortable with silence and by listening. It may take more than one meeting in a relaxed atmosphere for the patient to feel comfortable. Listening to patients, giving them time and paying attention to the patients' reactions to the information all help them understand what was told to them. This leads to shared decision-making, and the patient can then participate in her treatment with a better understanding of the situation.

A medical student I worked with described a meaningful and positive interaction she witnessed. Here it is, in Danielle Mascarenas's own words:

A year later (present day), his primary doctor and wife urged him again to see the renal specialists, who again suggested that he get a kidney biopsy. During a talk about the benefits and risks of a biopsy, I could see the patient obviously becoming uneasy with beads of sweat developing on his forehead. He was visibly anxious by the discussion and I could tell that my resident noticed this as well. The resident stopped mid-discussion, put his hand on his shoulder and asked the patient what was bothering him. The patient's eyes began to tear up as he said with a shaky voice that he was "deathly afraid of the complications" and could not "stand to think about what would happen to his wife and nine-year-old daughter if something went wrong." The resident paused and let the patient express his concerns. He listened closely and when the patient finished, the resident repeated back what he understood. The patient nodded in agreement and then the resident proceeded to address each issue/fear thoroughly. He did such a great job explaining and educating the patient that I could tell the patient was becoming more at ease throughout the conversation. It was also interesting to see how the resident discussed these worries without bias and without trying to persuade the patient to do something—he was simply educating. When he was done, the resident suggested the patient go home and think about what they discussed that day. He wanted him to make his own decision, and he supplied him with the knowledge he needed to do so. It was an inspiring encounter.

And here is a description from Zachary Gillooly, who was working in pediatrics. It is inspiringly positive.

The patient's parents were from Mexico and spoke very little English. The attending physician on the service very politely sat the parents down in a neutral room, with an interpreter, and went over every detail of the patient's diagnosis, treatment, and prognosis.

Consider the scenario of a patient who has tried several treatments for a cancer that is difficult to treat in most cases, and this patient has had no benefit from the previous treatments. Suppose that there is a report in a prominent medical journal that states that 10 percent of patients had an improvement in their disease from a new treatment. The report goes on to say that the improvement lasts for about three months. The report also describes the side effects of the treatment and its costs. The patient meets with his doctor to discuss what should be done at this point. There are many possible ways the discussion could proceed. Here are two examples of how the new treatment could be presented to the patient.

One doctor could say, "We have a new treatment I read about in a journal. It showed that 10 percent of patients had benefit from this treatment that was developed by a major medical center. Do you want to try it?" The patient may just focus on "10 percent benefit" and say, "Let's try it." The decision is made, and plans are put in place to start this treatment.

Another doctor might say, "This is a difficult situation. We need to discuss this in detail. We have to talk about keeping you comfortable and allowing you to spend time at home with your family. However, I did read a report in a journal recently. The report says 10 percent of patients had improvement. But nine out of ten patients did not have any benefit. The benefit in those who did improve lasted for three or so months. The treatment did cause some nausea and vomiting. Some patients got numbness of their hands, and others got some lung damage. The treatment is not covered by insurance and may cost you and your family about $20,000."

The two conversations show two extremes that may occur when different doctors meet different patients. The differences in the depth of the discussion make it more likely that the first patient will agree to the new treatment because only one side of the issue was presented. The second patient might make the same decision, but it would be an informed decision—which is the right thing.

Why this difference in the depth and detail of these two scenarios? The reasons are complex and are explored further in chapters 8 through 10 on the reasons why doctors over-treat. As discussed in chapter 1, there is an element of denial on the part of the provider, or, as some have suggested, there is some degree of self-delusion. What ends up occurring is a piecemeal perception on the doctor's part of what is happening to the patient and also what can be done to correct the problem. The doctor thinks only of one side of the disease and treatment. The doctor's self-deception leads to her presenting an unbalanced picture. She may explain the situation to the patient but with a bias. Although the physician may even explain the statistics, subconsciously she creates a mental filter and thus only presents information that goes along with her thinking. It is more common for doctors to present information that sounds "positive." The picture the patient gets is over-optimistic. It is likely such a doctor will convince patients to undertake more treatments, rather than fewer, and focus on treatment of the disease, rather than considering the patient's welfare and comfort.

In other words, the physician may give false hope rather than a realistic picture. Brown argues that such optimism is always harmful if it rests on the patient's ignorance of his disease prognosis.[13] She encourages the patient to work out his treatment decisions in a way that is concordant with his values, but with the requirement that this evaluation be fully informed and not the result of confusion or ignorance.

Understanding hope, positive thinking and acceptance of reality is not easy. It is very individual, and each person reacts differently. But it is clear that honest conversation is necessary if patients are to make decisions that give them the best chance of achieving their own realistic goals.

Hope and optimism are helpful in dealing with difficult situations. They give us a reason to try to fix the problems we face. But when it is clear that given the situation we are facing, the treatments available for our disease are not going to help us, we need to face the reality. This is where good communication becomes critical. Facing the reality of our serious illness helps us deal with the situation and thereby find the best solution, even if it is not what we had hoped for. Doctors often fail to provide this.

Hope is a feeling that we all require to cope with bad situations. Hope is an important way of dealing with difficulties of all kinds. When faced with financial loss, a failing personal relationship or a serious illness, life-changing or life-threatening, we cling to hope. The stock market may crash, but my company will survive. My spouse may be difficult, but we can rebuild our marriage. My illness will be mild; the medical condition can be fixed or at least controlled. Without that feeling of hope, we would not be able to survive the crisis. Hope in itself is not denial. But at some point, a transition needs to be made. Reality has to be accepted. In the setting of a serious medical situation, the responsibility for this transition to reality lies with the medical professionals who have the relevant knowledge and expertise. They must provide clear information. You as the patient can get a better understanding by asking questions or trying to inform yourself by reading or talking to other people.

But hope must give way to acceptance of reality—not to take away all hope, but to provide hope appropriate to the circumstances. (Your spouse may have left you, but you have friends; you have a life, and it could be a good life.)

With medical problems the impact may occur in multiple steps or may happen suddenly and catastrophically. An athlete diagnosed with rheumatoid arthritis has to face reality differently from someone who is paralyzed after a motor vehicle crash. In each situation, the conversation, the hope and the reality will be different: trials with treatments and waiting to see how well they work; consideration of various steps in the rehabilitation program and how the person adjusts to the process. The conversation will change as time goes on. Hope of response to the treatment will need to be adjusted to the reality of how well the arthritis is controlled, how severe the side effects of the treatment are. Acceptance of the reality of the paralysis becomes the focus of the patient's adaptation to the new loss of function.

Hope and reality need to go hand in hand, and honesty and openness are required at all the different stages of the physical and emotional changes that occur as time goes on. For most people, conveying bad news is not easy, but medical professionals must do this to help the patient cope with the problem and receive the best outcome and the maximum comfort.

Studies have shown that when the doctors speak clearly and use honest phrases like "You will not be able to compete in a tournament" or "You will need oxygen for the rest of your life," patients are able to deal with their situation more easily. Use of vague euphemisms like "Things may not go too well" just delay the adjustment to reality. Discussion should include, as appropriate, words like "death" and "disability." Even with clear statements regarding the serious illness, hope can be maintained—hope for support, hope for adjustment and hope for comfort at time of death. False hope, given by use of soft phrases or by evading the truth, is harmful to the patient. Hope and false hope are not the same. *False hope does not help anyone.*

Teneille Brown states that encouraging false hope is always unduly harmful if it rests on the patient's ignorance of his disease prognosis.[14] She urges the patient to work this out in a way that is concordant with his values, but with the requirement that this evaluation be fully informed and not the result of confusion or ignorance.

Information regarding the patient's condition and the chances of good outcome or bad must be stated truthfully. When new, alternative and even "long-shot" treatments are discussed, the explanation must be detailed and complete and include the expected outcomes. After failure of the initial treatment with the standard process that works for most patients, alternative treatments should be discussed. Even the "standard" treatment should be discussed fully. How long is the benefit likely to last? What are the side effects? These are core issues, and each needs to be expanded depending on the circumstances. When doctor and patient are faced with failure of the best treatment, the discussion becomes more critical. More details are required for the patient to make an *informed* decision. The patient needs to learn all that is known about the next treatment. Does it just control the disease, or does it have a good chance of making the patient function or feel better? If there is benefit from the treatment, how long is it expected to last—a short time or for a meaningful period?

There are many details that the doctor must provide. As the patient, you must ask questions and get a clear understanding of the likely outcomes, treatments available and how effective they are. Chapter 5, "Planning for Your Life, Illness and Death," provides a more detailed list of questions to ask. One way to decide if a treatment that is offered is right for you is to find out what the best possible outcome would be. Find out if the "best" will make you feel better or make you live longer. If the "best" is an improvement in a test or X-ray without making you feel better, you may not think the treatment is worthwhile. The acceptance of the best must also take into account how often that "best" result happens. If the "best" occurs only in one out of 20 cases, you may rethink taking the offered treatment.

The patient should be the center of the whole encounter—this should not be forgotten. In the August 2, 2010, issue of *The New Yorker*, surgeon Atul Gawande describes several instances of physicians who could not deal with the reality that the treatments they tried had not worked.[15] Rather than sitting down with the patient and the family to discuss the situation honestly, they chose to talk about another possible treatment that *might* work. The discussion did not include the chances of success or even, if successful, how long the benefit would last. The patient's overall status was not the focus of the discussion; the physicians were only trying to address the immediate issue. The reasons why doctors fail to look at the patient as a whole and become too focused on a disease or immediate problem are addressed in more detail in chapter 8.

The title of Gawande's article is "Letting Go." The patient and family and the medical personnel have a hard time letting go. They cannot let go of their false hope. It is a complex issue and will be discussed further on in this book.

Part of good communication means that the doctor recognizes the patient's need for clear and detailed information, starting with the basic use of language. Doctors are trained in an environment of technical terms (often of Greek or Latin origin), abbreviations and sometimes cryptic, incomplete sentences. They are so used to this way of speaking with their colleagues that they do not even realize how puzzling this language can be to patients. If the doctor uses technical terms for the explanation of your problem, the treatment choices and the expectations from the treatment, do not hesitate to say, "I do not understand what that means." Discussing treatment choices and outcomes requires detailed explanations, with clear formulation of chances of benefit and harm. What can I expect without treatment? What can I expect if the treatment is successful and if it is not?

We all have a built-in psychological bias toward hearing and remembering optimistic information. Research by neurobiologists has found that good news is processed differently from bad news by the brain. Some of the ways in which this manifests in our behavior have been summarized by Brown.[16] First we think we have more control over circumstances than we actually do. One example is that many of us believe that if we, ourselves, throw the dice in a game of chance, we will come out ahead. Similarly, we think we will do better than others, be it on job prospects or escaping injury in a motor vehicle crash. We transpose these feelings to medical situations. We think that we will do better than others and that even if we have a bad disease, things will get better. We convince ourselves that the statistics apply to "others."

Denial is a complex, poorly understood phenomenon—but it is real.

During their training, doctors are taught how to *get* information *from* patients. Starting early in medical school, they practice this regularly and become good at it. Unfortunately in our system, little training is given about how to *give* information *to* patients. Explaining the disease and the treatment options in understandable language is not a regular part of a doctor's training. Giving bad news is more difficult, and unfortunately training in that has been grossly neglected. This situation is improving, and many medical schools now incorporate this skill into the curriculum.

Here is a quote from a young doctor after she had met with a patient.

What I lacked in my encounter with Mrs. K was mastery of that self-reflective process. As an average physician-in-training, I had empathy, but the mark of a good physician is the manner of conveying that empathy. In between my examining and advising had I stopped to reflect, perhaps I could have made that connection. Perhaps I could have noticed how little room I had left for Mrs. K's questions. That pause of breath in a string of medical interrogation. That moment of opportune silence that can be filled with thought, emotion, concern, is not something I can measure.[17]

How do we convey the reality of a bad situation? This and related questions require explaining "odds" or in technical terms, "statistics." Statistics can be tricky, as chapter 7 explains. But the doctor needs to explain to patients what can happen: the different possible results and what is more or less likely. It has been said that a good medical decision reflects the patient's values, applies scientific evidence, considers medical expertise and acknowledges uncertainty. This is not an easy combination, but the doctor should help you as the patient strive toward it.

Another simple communication tool is for doctors to draw out patients—ask what they understand, ask how they feel. Asking about hopes, goals and reality opens up communication. Communication is a two-way process. The doctor must give information to the patient. But the patient must have a chance to think and understand the information. Afterwards the patient must have time to express his feelings and concerns, and, of course, an opportunity to ask questions. If everyone is on the same page, it is helpful to all.

What I have described relates to all types of medical encounters. It applies to most types of diseases, including those that have a good chance of being controlled or cured. We will now look deeper at more difficult situations, when communication is more challenging.

Unfortunately, situations arise when the best available treatments and lifestyle modifications do not work. At such times, the patient and doctor are dealing with changes—change in expected outcome, change in needed treatment, change in the life of the patient. These are difficult to deal with. Both parties have to modify their thinking and adjust to the new reality.

The patient's response to this situation can be one of acceptance, denial or hope—or a combination of all of these. Here we will discuss and analyze how medical professionals react to these cases. In most, the doctors respond the same way they reacted before: they explain the problem, discuss options and provide hope. Hope as appropriate to the situation, but not false hope. At that point, trial of another treatment or promise of providing the best supportive care to offer comfort can be considered. Some providers are not able to deal with the options too well. They cannot give bad news. They try to divert the conversation to other issues. They avoid the discussion, with the belief that the truth will hurt, and they try to cover it up. They use euphemisms. This reflects a combination of their own discomfort with the reality and their fear of the patient's reaction. Another complicating factor is that there are often multiple doctors taking care of the patient. Each may think that one of the others has had the conversation.

Like most of us, doctors want to think of the positive; they want to be optimistic. One factor that gives them optimism is the success of previous patients. Even if the chances of improving the condition of the patient in front of him are small, the doctor may remember a previous case that, despite the odds, did well. That exceptional case gives the doctor hope, and he may pass that hope on to the patient. The odds remain against any benefit to the patient, but the shared optimism can drive decisions and actions.

False optimism has another aspect. Patients and family members often hear about patients who were seriously ill and were given no chance of recovery but recovered nonetheless. These situations are fairly common. Stories from friends or the media make the patient optimistic. We hear of someone "who was given three months to live" and is doing well one year later. However, when looked into in detail, most often it turns out that the patient in the story was different from our patient or that the so-called "three months" was an average number, and all averages have a range. Projections from anecdotes or the media are usually irrelevant or are taken out of context, and you must be careful before applying the information to yourself. The same needs to be emphasized regarding new treatments or "breakthroughs," even those reported in respected medical journals. The media hype the benefits of new treatments, and the Internet is full of news of "cures," news that has not been subjected to any sort of critical inspection. Physicians must scrutinize all these pieces of information carefully before applying them to the patient at hand. If you as a patient or family member read about a treatment that might be relevant to you, discussing this information with your doctor should clarify the issue.

Doctors often feel that they are compelled by the patient or the family to provide treatments that are excessive or futile. Rather than explain and discuss the reality, they may just go ahead and do what the patient requests. This is not really in the patient's best interest, because it is based on a false premise. Unfortunately, the doctors are dealing with the patient's false hopes. These hopes are raised by the hype, overstatement and misunderstanding of the progress made in medical research and treatment. For example, certain types of lung cancer can now be treated with less toxic and more effective drugs. Cures are still rare. These successes are with small sub-groups of patients. But patients hear that lung cancer can be put into remission for some period of time. The specifics of this progress are hard to understand. The media just write about the progress in the treatment of "lung cancer." This causes a lot of confusion. When patients ask for treatments based on incomplete information, it is the doctor's responsibility to clarify the facts. This takes time, and it is difficult. Some doctors take the easy way out and just go ahead and start the treatment.

In summary, communication—honest and complete—between doctors and patients is essential for the good and appropriate care of every patient. It is more difficult when the illness is severe; yet that is the time when it is needed most. Doctors have an obligation to provide full and honest information.

3

Religion, Healing and Death

When faced with serious illness or death, patients and their loved ones need solace, comfort and understanding. Their faith, their religion, their belief system all play a role in providing these. One of the purposes of religion is to guide the living through the experience of death.

Religion, healing and death have been linked at least as far back as we have archeological evidence.[1] Many archeologists think that cave paintings, monoliths and temples started as responses to death. These were attempts to understand, ward off or reduce the impact of death on the dying person and on those still alive. Further, in many ancient cultures, the priests were also the first healers. Because the priests were powerful, had leadership qualities and were the persons to whom the public came in times of difficulty, they sought to explain to themselves and to the laity the mysteries of the world. Death could have been considered the ultimate mystery. Belief systems and religion provided collective comfort from various terrors, including death. Religion became an active expression of a sense of belonging and throughout history has provided solace to many.

In different cultures and locations, religion took different directions, evolving into varied mythologies and beliefs with corresponding practices. Some believed, as their priests said, that the soul was not really dead and would migrate from the body of the dead person to that of another living being. Others believed in eternal rest until the Day of Judgment, and so on. Forms of disposal of the dead body could be related to these beliefs. Those who believed in eternal life and those who believed in the Day of Judgment buried the dead in an intact form. Those who believed in the transmigration of the soul cremated the remains. Leaders (religious and secular) presided over death rituals where they consoled those left behind. In societies where war was a way of life, there were many deaths, and many families needed solace and an explanation for the problems they faced.

The consoling rituals that are common after death are often based on religion and are helpful to those who knew and loved the deceased. These rituals vary from place to place and are different for each group. Deep emotions associated with religion may be expressed publicly through art, music and dance. They are comforting to believers and non-believers, as they reflect human feelings and help people to connect with each other, especially in difficult times. They create a sense of belonging, whether through chanting, prayer or eulogies. Some groups celebrate the life of the person; others mourn the death. In some cultures, display of grief is the norm, and in others mourning is silent. Some set a specific period for intense mourning, such as the Jewish custom of sitting shiva for seven days. There is no right or wrong approach. The practices are based on traditions, culture and the faith of the person or community. The important point is that rituals help to bring closure, and they help the living to deal with and accept the reality of death. The virtually universal existence of rituals at death suggests that most societies recognize the reality of death; yet some people are not able to accept that death is inevitable.

Through their role at the time of death, religious leaders historically have had a significant degree of control over rituals; mourning—its demonstration, its duration—could be dictated by them. In addition, we must remember that illness is common before death. The priests thus interacted with the ill and their families before someone died. As medical knowledge advanced, some people lived longer. In some cases, priests were credited with the healing. The priests later gained the authority to tell the laity when to accept medical treatments and when to accept death. The interpretation of such dictates has varied and has been modified regularly; now there are multiple statements interpreted in different ways, making it difficult for dying patients and their families to decide when to accept death as part of the natural order of life and when to resist the dying process.

Personal faith is a strong force. Most people cannot define their faith, but nevertheless it gives them comfort; it allows them to rise above and go beyond the immediate problem, and it provides consolation.

For some, thinking about the meaning of life is a way of obtaining solace. Others get help from their own belief systems. These also are individual. Whatever his or her professed faith, each person has a unique belief system. It may be based on science, religion, philosophy or none of these. Belief systems allow people to deal with the situation they face. Again, the belief system is personal; it is often not definable, but it provides understanding and acceptance.

Religion is a common way to derive solace. By using religion, many people get what they need at the time of crisis and difficulty. Religion has a structure that helps the person. The priests, nuns and temple leaders all are trained to give help to people in need. Religious organizations have hospital chaplains and volunteers who can talk to people in distress and provide help. Religious teachings that people may have been exposed to in the course of their lives offer a way for dealing with a difficult situation. Religious stories and parables add to the understanding of one's situation and allow one to realize that he or she is not alone.

I was talking to Joan Gibson, a hospital chaplain and ethicist. She said that the nuns she worked with at a particular Catholic hospital were sympathetic toward dying patients. Their focus was the spiritual comfort of those who were dealing with death or serious illness. At the time of death, these nuns did not emphasize the doctrine of the Catholic Church but gave spiritual comfort. Most religious professionals provide consolation and comfort, though there are some exceptions.

Even within the same religion, writings may not be consistent regarding continuing medical treatments when the end of life is near and certain. My experience with Hindu and Navajo families is one of individual choices; in these traditions there is no written or stated uniform pronouncement for either point of view. This is also true of the dominant religions in the United States. The one clear statement I did find from a dominant American religion was from Pope John Paul II when he spoke to a group of visiting doctors at the Vatican. He said, "It is thus necessary to approach the ill with that healthy realism which avoids generating, in those who suffer, the illusion of medicine's omnipotence," and "In this perspective, extreme measures at all costs, even with the best of intentions, would be, in the end, not only useless, but not fully respectful to the patient."[2] The pope clearly stated that accepting death is the right course of action.

I have used three terms in this section—"faith," "belief system" and "religion." These words are difficult to define, and it is hard to separate them from each other. "Spirituality" is another such term. Some have defined spirituality as a way of dealing with the "larger" issues like the meaning and purpose of life. Whether or not one believes in the existence of a deity, some people get comfort through spirituality. Without trying to separate these ways of dealing with a bad situation, it is important to understand that each person is different. Leaders from time immemorial have understood the need for comfort and solace. They have provided different ways of achieving this peace; each person adapts these tools to his or her circumstance. Having flexibility and adaptability has helped humanity from the dawn of civilization. From the Stone Age, Bronze Age and Iron Age through the civilizations of China, India and ancient Greece to the present, this has been so. Religious leaders have filled an essential need in this context. Compassionate action is the heart of religious expression.

Religious leaders and groups have a major impact on the lives of many people. The response to death and serious illness is influenced strongly by the patient's and family's beliefs about religion, God and spirituality. Just as with religious people, nonreligious people are also influenced by their beliefs—whatever they may be. The spectrum of beliefs is wide, and within each category there are differences. When it comes to dealing with serious illness and death, the reactions, even among believers, vary. Some devout Catholics, for example, accept Pope John Paul II's point about the limits of medicine and will allow the patient to die comfortably. Others feel that medical treatments should be continued until death. Similar discrepancies and variations occur among people of different faiths and even among those who call themselves a-religious or nonreligious; medical providers and patients and families should keep this in mind. In fact, when making decisions about serious medical problems, it helps to discuss and acknowledge religious beliefs openly.

In the context of serious illness and death, religion plays a major role. One is the role to console, accept and even celebrate the life of the dying person. Among my most moving experiences has been listening to the singing of beautiful religious songs by the family of a woman with leukemia. The patient and family had tried the best treatments available. Once it was clear that no further treatments would help, they accepted that the end was near. The extended circle of family and friends came to the hospital and surrounded the bed, held hands and wept. They sang non-stop for about a day and a half, one of the most beautiful songs I have heard. The patient died in comfort, and the family had closure. In a positive and a consoling way, faith helped the family and the patient. She died with faith, courage and acceptance.

I have worked with many patients and families who did not accept medical reality. They did not accept that death was near. Some were influenced by their faith and religion. (They believed in different gods and had varying degrees of faith.) They felt that their faith would make them recover, that their God would provide a "miracle cure." After acknowledging their faith, we went on to a further discussion on the nature of the disease, treatments that had already been tried and did not help, and how, despite the best treatment, the disease was progressing. Most often this helped them accept that comfort care was in the patients' best interest. Patients who were not religious also denied medical reality. Explanation, answering their questions and concerns, did in many cases lead to acceptance. In early Catholic literature there is a road map for the death bed called *ars moriendi*. It states in part, "The brave person did not battle Death, but regarded dying as a test of one's trust in God, an earthly purification to be followed by heavenly rewards, a sacred rite of passage."[3]

Accepting death and making the time before death peaceful and comforting is one of the best gifts we can give to ourselves, our family and our loved ones. It does happen, but far too often people suffer before they die because there is denial of reality.

Writing on the role of the physician, Pope Paul VI said, "The physician's duty consists rather of endeavoring to soothe the suffering instead of prolonging as long as possible by any means and under any conditions a life that is naturally approaching its conclusion."[4]

Denial and lack of acceptance of death occur because of many forces in our society. One factor (discussed in chapter 9) is the medical community. But another major reason is the misguided use of religion by a small group of people who claim that religion and God "require" that one must continue treatments in all circumstances regardless of the biological reality. It is not possible to categorize this group with a label except to say that some of them state that they speak from their faiths. At times, they invoke "God," but many do not identify themselves further.

Paradoxically, these activists cause difficulties for patients and families in two opposite ways. Some have persuaded patients and families not to take treatments for illnesses that are easily treatable, leading to tragic outcomes. Some have persuaded parents not to immunize their children, thus endangering not just their own families but also the community at large, as occurred with the measles outbreak in early 2015.[5]

In the context of serious illness and patients who have diseases for which there is no reasonable treatment, some religious extremists have spread the false idea that doctors deliberately withhold treatment from patients. They have stated that doctors do not respect patients or their wishes, stop treatments too soon and let patients die. They accuse the physicians of ulterior motives (such as ageism, racism or financial incentives) for stopping treatments. They often contradict themselves, as I will point out. These groups are a mix of people with no clear unifying feature except that they do not trust the medical profession.

As stated above, some oppose well-established treatments while others want patients to continue treatments when it is clear that the treatment will only cause pain and suffering. These misguided people have political support and have succeeded in persuading some politicians to enact laws that override medical judgment and force physicians to treat patients when no treatment is reasonable. Instead of being compassionate, as religious teachings tell us we should be, they cause more difficulties for patients and doctors.

Sometimes the problem is complicated by the belief that illness is a divine punishment for some wrongdoing. Myrick C. Shinall Jr., a surgeon and a religious scholar at Vanderbilt University in Nashville, has looked into the role of religion in acceptance of pain and suffering before death. In a 2014 article he wrote, "Among Christians, one explanation for preference for aggressive, life prolonging care is the influence of the idea of martyrdom, which became the normative form of dying in early Christianity."[6]

Shinall points out that words influence actions, and vice versa—the discourse of death is shaped by the discourse of martyrdom. He suggests that the deaths of martyrs were, in a sense, recapitulating the death of Christ. He points out that illness and other types of physical pain are often described as "my cross to bear."

He reminds us of some of the other common phrases we use when referring to illness and treatment of diseases—the metaphors of combat. We talk about our "*war* on cancer," "*fighting* off infections," "*battling* serious illness," "*bombarding* cancer with radiation." In a sense, we transform deaths from disease into violent ends.

Martyrdom was attained by only a few, but metaphorically it affects the thinking of many facing death due to illness. It is seen as a way to face (painful) death with courage and faith in God. A decision to pursue or continue life-prolonging therapy may be a faith-inspired decision to undergo pain.

Christopher Meyers is a professor of philosophy at California State University in Bakersfield. He has made some observations and commented on the role of religious beliefs and how they affect decisions made by seriously ill people. He states that religious beliefs are a dominant factor for many patients and families facing life-threatening illness.[7] He has noted that medical providers generally honor these beliefs. He further states that religious pronouncements made by patients and families should not be given a blanket waiver. Doctors should at least challenge such statements and make sure that such pronouncements are coherent and internally consistent. Religious beliefs should not be exempt from challenge just because they are religious. He cites a situation where a family member who claimed he was religious wanted his dying mother to be treated aggressively because he believed God would intervene. He also wanted the doctors not to give pain medications because that would "interfere with God's actions." This, to me, brings in a bigger question: the balance between conscience and faith. Did the son have compassion for his mother? How could his conscience allow her to suffer? Meyers goes on to say that the doctor's primary responsibility is to the person in the bed. In the case above, the son's statements were internally inconsistent. Meyers also explains that some family members use a religious argument because they understand that doctors will usually not challenge a religious argument. Some families use the hope for a miracle as a trump card. If they say they are waiting for a miracle, it is very difficult for the providers to counter that statement.

Teneille Brown has analyzed this problem and also has given many useful suggestions. She suggests that medical students and doctors should be taught the importance of discussing such arguments with sensitivity and open communication.[8] This would allow them to refute irrational religious arguments. It often helps to bring clergy into the discussion, because they can explain the religious perspective to the patient and family and may be trusted by the family.

This mind-set, this emphasis on painful medical treatments with tubes and machines, is of no value. Death is inevitable, and its acceptance serves everyone well. These proponents of aggressive treatments to the end—whatever their agenda, whatever their thinking—are causing pain and suffering. It appears that they believe, in some fashion, that humans are immortal or at least that divine intervention can make a terminally ill patient well again, and that this can be achieved if the patient and family have strong enough faith, pray fervently and accept every possible treatment, however unpleasant and however slim the chances of success. What is important to understand is that such groups and some members of these groups cause considerable harm to patients and their families. One of the leaders of this movement is Wesley J. Smith.

Smith is a lawyer who advocates from a religious perspective. It is difficult to determine if he represents a particular group or if his advocacy comes from his own thinking. Smith has stated many times, including in his book *Culture of Death: The Assault on Medical Ethics in America* and in a blog posting, "Futile Care Theory: Bioethicists Should Stop Pretending They Are Doing Patients a Favor," that physicians must continue life-sustaining treatments if the patient wants them.[9] He states that doctors should not have authority to stop a treatment even when it is only prolonging the process of dying.

Smith strongly objects to attempts by doctors to have control over the use of futile treatments. He does not seem to understand that the assessment of whether or not a treatment will help or hurt a patient can only be made on the basis of medical expertise. This requires understanding the meaning of each test and how the patient reacted to previous treatments, as well as the patient's underlying health status. Medical knowledge and experience are essential for guiding decisions regarding treatments. It takes a competent and caring physician to decide whether a proposed or ongoing treatment will help to achieve the patient's medical goals or is futile.

As an aside, I would like to point out a contradiction by Smith. He has stated in other blogs that doctors want to stop such treatments because they want to save money. Yet in *Culture of Death,* he states that "Intensive Care Units were major profit centers for hospitals."[10] In a more recent blog, he said:

Medical futility disputes often involve the question of harming the patient. Family/ patient believe they should decide what constitutes "harm" in these cases, and that for the patient/family, the greatest harm would be death. Hence, they insist that efficacious treatment to extend life continue—as the way to avoid harm. That is, after all, a fundamental purpose of medicine when staying alive is wanted. Bioethicists and some doctors believe that they get to decide what constitutes "harm." Thus, if a patient is unlikely to recover or even lead a "meaningful" life, they insist on being able to stop wanted treatment. Religion is also a large factor in many of these situations. The secularist view sees suffering as the worst harm; many religions, particularly more traditional approaches to Catholicism, Islam, and Judaism, death. Thus, forcing treatment to cease is often viewed as disrespecting freedom of religion. At the same time, many futilitarians believe in judging "harm" on the macro level. They look beyond the patient to perceived emotional harm to the family—and the morale of the reluctant medical team—as well as financial harm to society by "investing" resources on the patient supposedly more wisely spent elsewhere.[11]

I disagree with Wesley Smith. As I have shown in my quotations from two popes and from articles in the *Lancet* described below, comfort before death and acceptance of medical reality has been supported by all major religions. I do agree with Smith when he states, "Education and continual mediation should be the watchword." Also, I agree with him that the doctors should be frank about the consequences of continuing treatments. (Yes, treatments can cause harmful effects, but "care" helps the patient.)

Here is a statement on the issue by the Catholic Health Association (CHA), which provides policy guidance to the church's 600 hospitals and 1,400 long-term care facilities in the United States:

But the unprecedented science and technology available to us today cannot change one fact of life: There comes a time when death is inevitable. Science may be able to force air into a dying person's lungs or pump nutrients into the digestive system. In short, science can prolong the dying process. But is that really what we want from our healthcare system?

The question our society must confront is: Should healthcare professionals be required to use technology to prolong a dying patient's life when those interventions violate longstanding medical ethics and standards, while providing no relief or benefit to the patient?

In striving for the proper balance, we must ask ourselves some key questions: How much care is the right amount of care? When do healthcare interventions— in the form of machinery and technology—become inhumane rather than heroic? What, in fact, is a death with dignity? These questions are deeply personal, and that's why we will continue to urge all individuals to state their end-of-life wishes through an advance directive or a healthcare proxy. But these very personal decisions are now becoming a societal issue as well—one that will confront physicians and families again and again in the years to come.[12]

Wesley Smith took issue with the CHA's position in his May 10, 2010, blog. I think the CHA's statements are sensible and should be discussed and followed.

Doctors should discontinue futile interventions when it is clear that they are not helping the patient and are causing distress and harm. A medical treatment should be used only when medically indicated and appropriate. Attitudes of people like Smith hurt patients and their families by prolonging the agony and depriving patients of a chance to say their goodbyes and achieve spiritual peace.

Smith should pay heed to what Pope John Paul II said.

When it is clear that medical treatments have failed, when no medical interventions can lead to recovery from a serious illness, the patient should be allowed to die in peace. It is our responsibility as families and health-care providers to prevent such pernicious ideas as Wesley Smith's from becoming a barrier to a comfortable death. Religion should help to provide solace and comfort. It should not lead to distress.

In 2005 the *Lancet*, a medical journal published in England, ran a series of seven articles on religion and the end of life.[13] Appearing in successive weekly issues, these articles covered Hindu, Islamic, Jewish, Buddhist, traditional Christian, Catholic and secular humanistic points of view. Each article was written by a scholar of that religion from a major university in England or the United States. They describe the general tenets of each religion and their understanding and beliefs regarding their God.

These articles point out that there are different views on the meaning of life and the relationship to a supreme being. These differences are notable among the different religions. But importantly within each group there are different approaches to what patients and families should do when faced with serious illness and death. Some say that life is precious and must be preserved as long as possible by whatever means possible, but in each religion there is also a strong voice that says that death is a part of life and must be accepted. This will allow peace and tranquility, and if you believe in a God, it is the way to give yourself to the Supreme Power. There are many who advocate acceptance of death. They acknowledge that there are limits to what medicine can do. There are strong statements from each religion that there is no justification to "prolong life at all cost." Nor is there a justification to demand treatments that the medical profession considers to be futile. It is worth noting that the Christian Medical and Dental Association issued an ethics statement asserting that if "medical treatment prolongs pain and suffering and postpones the moment of death . . . it may then be appropriate for a patient with decision-making capacity to refuse medical interventions."[14]

In summary, the mainstream thought from all major religions is that acceptance of death is the best way to achieve union with their respective deities and provide dignity at life's end.

In a study of patients with advanced cancer from a hospital affiliated with Harvard Medical School, it was found that when medical teams provided spiritual support to patients, they were more likely to accept comfort care, use hospice services and die peacefully with their loved ones around them.[15] Tristram Engelhardt and Ana Smith Ilitis, while discussing the traditional Christian view in the *Lancet* series cited above, also emphasize the importance of discussing the religious values of the individual patient to ensure they are taken into account when making decisions about end-of-life care and treatment.[16] Myrick Shinall, cited earlier, emphasizes that understanding what religious issues are at stake is a major step when medical professionals are developing plans for care at the end of life.

A good death is one where the patient is comfortable, in comfortable surroundings. The family and friends are with the patient. They have a chance to say their goodbyes and can tell the patient they love and will miss him or her. The appropriate, compassionate religious professionals can help in achieving this goal.

4

Patient Autonomy and Medical Expertise

How to Find a Balance

For a long time, doctors told the patient what needed to be done, what they would do—and patients just accepted that. "You have an ulcer, and we will remove part of your stomach." There was no explanation, no discussion, and patients were not given options.

Gradually, starting in the 1970s, the tide turned. Medical professionals and society as a whole agreed that patients must be a party to the decision-making and that they have a right to full information about risks and benefits. The Patient Self-Determination Act (PSDA), a series of laws, was passed in the early 1990s by the federal government and most states.[1] Under these laws, medical providers were required to give the patient details of the disease, the proposed treatment and the expected results. The patient was to be fully informed and only then give, or withhold, permission to undergo the tests and treatments.

As we have seen, despite this many physicians do not give all the information the patient needs to make an informed decision. Still, the situation is better than it was before these laws were enacted. The most important point is that all adults have the right to refuse treatment. Treatment cannot be forced on us. If the patient lacks decision-making capacity (e.g., due to brain injury or advanced Alzheimer's disease), the person he designated in an advance directive acts on his behalf. If the patient has not chosen a surrogate, the law has defined a hierarchy in the family as to who will be the surrogate.

The freedom of choice available to us in the wake of the PSDA was a distinct improvement over the previous norm when patients were given no choices.

However, this autonomy has led to an unforeseen consequence that has caused tension between patients and medical providers. Many have interpreted this change to mean that patients can *demand* tests and treatments even if their providers feel these are not going to help and may even harm them. As an example, it is common for patients with back pain of a mild nature and short duration to ask for a magnetic resonance image (MRI) of their backs, although it is very clear that most back pain results from muscle strain and is short-lived. An MRI will be of no help to the patient. Despite this, many physicians go ahead and order one, reasoning that it costs me (the doctor) nothing and the patient will be happier. This leads to a lot of waste. Granted, the procedure has no known side effects, but it still costs the patient's insurance plan and may involve a co-pay. Why not persuade the patient to wait to see if a combination of exercises and muscle relaxants will resolve the pain? This tension becomes more pronounced as the complexity of the illness increases, and it can cause significant conflict when the condition is life-changing or life-threatening.

The situation gets more serious if the patient demands a treatment that is not helpful or may even be harmful. (For example, fusing vertebrae can limit motion and in a substantial percentage of cases does not resolve back pain—in fact, may make it worse.) Patients often demand treatments because they "heard" about them from someone. Doctors do try to explain why a given treatment is not in the patient's best interest. Also, doctors have to follow medical guidelines and can refuse to provide a treatment that is judged inappropriate or harmful.

Unfortunately, in some situations, for a variety of reasons, many physicians agree to provide such treatments. This is a complicated issue and is discussed in detail in chapters 8 through 10.

Another consequence of misunderstanding the meaning of autonomy is that some doctors give the patient options without any advice, comment or opinion. They think they are giving "neutral" information. We all need the doctor's help—even we physicians do when we fall ill ourselves. The doctors must provide us with information and options but should then give their opinion and recommendation about which option is better and why. This expert input is applicable in day-to-day encounters for simple problems and more so for complex, serious issues. In his book *Patient Autonomy and the Ethics of Responsibility*, physician-philosopher Alfred I. Tauber states, "The simplistic view that physicians need only facilitate autonomous decision-making by providing patients with pertinent information about available options is not enough. They must help patients identify and understand their own values, select suitable options and to cope with fears and anxieties."[2] Striking the balance between autonomy and medical expertise is difficult. What is clear is that an excess of either does not satisfy or benefit anyone.

Communication and open discussion are the most important way to strike a balance and to get the best outcome. When dealing with an illness that is life-changing or life-threatening, the discussion and communication become even more critical. At the same time, finding a balance between patient autonomy and the physician's need to control the situation based on medical reality becomes more difficult and, at times, contentious. Patients may not fully recognize the limits of what medical treatments can offer. Their hopes for a good outcome may cloud their judgment. They or their families want recovery and good health. On the other hand, the medical team, after due deliberation and full evaluation of the medical condition, may want to stop treatments directed at the disease and allow for the most comfortable end of life for the patient.

A time may come when it is appropriate for the medical team to override the patient's request or demand for a particular treatment. This should happen only after the medical team has explained the medical reality to the patient and the family. After taking into account the medical facts, after evaluating the available treatments and after considering what treatments have been tried and failed, the medical team may conclude that no further treatments will help the patient—and may, in fact, only harm her. The decision to withhold or withdraw a treatment should be based solely on medical evaluation of the situation of that patient and that disease at that time. Social and economic issues should not affect the decision. If the medical assessment makes clear that no treatment will control the disease or make the patient feel better, the treatment should not be given regardless of whether the patient is young or old, rich or poor. If the patient and family agree that further treatment is not in the patient's interest, everyone is served well.

Withholding or withdrawing treatments against the patient's wishes is not pleasant, but in some cases it needs to be done. Some may object to this approach and call it domineering or even "rationing"; they feel that patients have a right to any treatment they want. Let us examine this argument and understand what it can lead to.

A medical treatment is provided by a professional—one who is trained to assess the disease and who has knowledge as to what works for that disease and what the risks and drawbacks are for particular categories of patients. That kind of experience and knowledge should not and cannot be ignored. An informed, thoughtful assessment by appropriately trained professionals has credibility. Yes, there are situations where there is uncertainty and the treatment may offer partial benefit or efficacy. Such situations, of course, need to be discussed, as explained in the section on honesty and open communication in chapter 2. But in cases where it is clear that no treatment would work, professional judgment cannot be disregarded—it must receive full credibility and strength.

Two examples may help to make the point. Infections of the upper respiratory tract, which are common and self-limiting, are caused by viruses. Viruses are not killed by antibiotics, which kill bacteria. Many patients ask for antibiotics for these infections. It is clearly not proper to give antibiotics for viral infections. Yes, doctors often do give antibiotics for viral infections just to placate the patient, but that is not good medical practice. Not only does it result in killing off the patient's "good" bacteria (e.g., those involved in digestion), it also leads to the development of antibiotic-resistant bacteria—a threat to everyone.

At the other end of the spectrum, consider a patient with metastatic lung cancer that has not responded to previous treatments. The cancer continues to grow in multiple vital organs. For whatever reasons, the family or patient request full life-support treatments. Such a patient should be given every needed comfort measure, but should not be treated actively for the cancer or with life support. The patient's hopes are understandable, but medical reality and judgment cannot and should not be overlooked. Active treatment should not be undertaken. If started, such treatments should be discontinued if they fail to achieve a good outcome. Another point to re-emphasize is, as discussed in chapters 8 through 10, that doctors are more likely to prescribe more, rather than less; so if they say "no further treatment will work," it makes sense to accept that.

Yes, patient autonomy is important for good medical care, but it has its limits. Physicians can and should exert control when that is essential to the best interest of the patient.

I would like to quote here a short piece I wrote in our medical school's magazine in 2011. It is, I think, worth pondering.

JUST A THOUGHT

When the ethicist said: Patients should have autonomy
They did not mean the patient becomes the doctor.

When the ethicist said: Patients must have freedom of choice
They did not mean that they choose as in a cafeteria.

When the ethicist said: Patients must have proper information
They did not mean that the textbook be given to them.

When the ethicist said: Patients must get a balanced opinion
They did not mean there would be no opinion.

What the ethicist said: The problem must be explained to the patient, the patient must understand the situation, and the doctor and patient must work as a team to make the best decision for the patient.

Abraham Lincoln said that there are no absolutes. All people must be treated fairly, but there are other factors to consider. Here are his own words from a speech he gave on June 28, 1857, in Springfield, Illinois, nearly four years before he became president:

> I think that the authors of that notable instrument [the Declaration of Independence] intended to include all men, but they did not mean to declare all men equal in all respects. They did not mean to say all men were equal in color, size, intellect, moral development or social capacity. They defined with tolerable distinctness in what they did consider all men created equal—equal in certain inalienable rights, among which are life, liberty, and the pursuit of happiness. This they said, and this they meant. They did not mean to assert the obvious untruth, that all were then actually enjoying that equality, or yet, that they were about to confer it immediately upon them. In fact, they had no power to confer such a boon. They meant simply to declare the right, so that the enforcement of it might follow as circumstances should permit.
>
> They meant to set up a standard maxim for free society which should be familiar to all: constantly looked to, constantly labored for, and even though never perfectly attained, constantly approximated, and thereby constantly spreading and deepening its influence and augmenting the happiness and value of life to all people, of all colors, everywhere.[3]

5

Planning for Your Life, Illness and Death

If we think about our life and death, even in a general way, we might understand that planning for our life before death is a useful process. Most of us do a lot of planning for our lives. We do financial planning, we plan for our and our children's education and we plan to see how we can get housing we can afford and will be comfortable in. For some reason, very few of us plan and think about how we would deal with serious illness. We do not like to think about the worst thing that can happen to us—an illness that changes our life or may cause our death. Any one of us can get sick; it may come suddenly or gradually and make us unable to do what we can and like to do now. It is not necessary to live in fear of illness, but we should think of how we would deal with an illness. As Pulitzer Prize–winning poet Vijay Seshadri notes, "How shocking the obvious can be/If you're not ready for it."[1]

Some illnesses are short-lived, have an easy treatment to fix the problem and allow us to go back to our usual lives. That is great. But some illnesses change our lives drastically. Giving some thought to how we would deal with those changes makes us better prepared to address them. Obviously, we do not know what will happen to us or when. Just thinking about general goals and strategies is helpful. We all make plans for other unexpected events. We have a plan for what to do if there is a fire in the house. We are prepared for other emergencies like prolonged failure of water supply or electricity if there is a major storm. Even a general plan for how we would deal with a serious illness is helpful. Just as we discuss our plan in case of a fire with the whole family, it is useful for the whole family to have a general understanding as to what would be the best way to deal with a serious illness among us. In fact, it is best if plans are made by the whole family for the whole family. Everyone's opinion and input is valuable.

Another way of phrasing the discussion about what you would like to do if you had a serious illness is to express your goals and values. Talk to your family and friends; tell them what you value most and ask them what they do. To some, the feeling and satisfaction that they tried every medical treatment to control their illness is very important no matter what the chance of success is. To others, it is most important that they spend the last stage of life in a way that they can interact with the family and be comfortable enough to do that without the burden of active medical interventions.

A two-way discussion of values and goals opens up many areas that we do not think about or talk about. By talking about open-ended issues like values and goals, we are forced to think about details we never considered. The initial idea that we must avail ourselves of all that modern medicine has to offer may change when we discuss the details with our family and friends. The discussion may raise questions like "How likely is it that I will benefit?" "How hard will the treatment be?" We may start thinking of alternatives that promise more comfort before death. We may question our preconceived ideas that medicine can do so much.

Thinking about your goals and values is an important step that will help you to achieve comfort before death.

If such a discussion is held before there is any illness, everyone will be better prepared, and the decision is likely to be more rational than emotional. Many of the decisions are easy. A fall leads to a broken bone; it will need to be fixed. An acute attack of bronchitis will require a visit to the doctor to get antibiotics. But suppose the bronchitis turns out to be something more serious and the shortness of breath turns out to be from a damaged heart valve? Input and explanation from your medical provider will be necessary to understand what the problem is, what can be done to treat it and how successful the treatment can be. Yes, you cannot plan for all the scenarios unless you have a clear picture of what illness could affect you. That can only come after a sickness happens. However, some general discussion can help you clarify your own thoughts and those of your family. The discussion you have with your family, and the thoughts you have as to how you want to proceed, will help you to understand your own values and theirs. It will make clear what your wishes are. If it turns out that your illness is serious, treatment is limited, and you may not return to a normal life, you will already have a framework into which you can put the problem. You will also have a better understanding of how to work with your doctor. You can explain to the doctor what you value most. You can work with the doctor, taking into account your values, your wishes and your goals and see how these fit with what the doctor has to offer.

Despite that, four out of five Americans do not prepare the necessary paperwork, in what is called an advance directive, to guide their physicians and families if they become so seriously ill that they themselves become incapable of expressing what they want.[2] On the other hand, 80 percent of doctors state in their own advance directives that "they have a striking personal preference to forego high intensity care for themselves at the end of life and prefer to die gently and naturally."[3] Philip A. Pizzo, former dean of the Stanford Medical School, and David M. Walker, former comptroller general of the United States, have confirmed this.[4]

We don't think of, and certainly don't discuss, how we would like to die. It is somewhere in the (remote) future. But what about those who have a serious illness? Why don't they think about how they would like to die? It has been said, half jokingly, that we think of death as being optional. The ex-husband of the editor who has helped me with this book had a serious chronic illness. He refused to make any plans for his illness and death because he said, "I will get better." He effectively ceded to others choices such as his living arrangements as his health declined. Her current husband and she have talked about their values and goals and have clear plans for their serious illnesses and deaths.

When people have not discussed their goals and values with their families, once they become seriously ill they often uses phrases like "I am a fighter; I want everything done." Unfortunately, because they have neither thought about the issues nor talked about them, they make these statements based on the prevailing norms of society. Our society respects those who try their best, which is fine. However, to try to do something that is not achievable can be counterproductive, even harmful. Those who have thought about the process of serious illness and death have a better understanding of the realities of life, illness and what medical science can and cannot do. With a thoughtful approach, we often avoid unhelpful, painful interventions.

In the community of La Crosse, Wisconsin, there is a clinic that is part of the Gundersen Lutheran Health System.[5] The clinic has worked with the community for many years and explained to the people the benefits of having discussions about their choices. The choices are respected; no one tries to persuade people to make choices one way or the other. The personnel help the community by telling them about the advantages of thinking about, talking about and writing down their choices. They are available to answer their questions when needed. As a result of this effort, over 90 percent of people in La Crosse have made their choices clear. Bud Hammes and Linda Briggs, employees of the Gundersen Clinic, have recently been awarded the Tribeca Fest Award for their work in promoting these advance directives.

Related to lack of discussion is the unfortunate occurrence of patients accepting painful treatments because their families wants them to "try their best." These may be treatments that are not supported by the doctors or wanted by the patients. In a crisis situation, because no discussion was held, the patient may agree to such treatments. This just adds more difficulties for all concerned. The decision to take or not to take a treatment should be made, as far as possible, by the patient.

If you hold such a discussion with your family ahead of time, in the extreme situation of an illness that has a low chance of beneficial treatment, or for which the suggested treatment is harsh, you as the patient will be in a better position to talk to the doctor and work out the best plan for *you*. If you have not thought about these issues, if you have not talked to your family about them, you will become a passive participant in dealing with your own illness. Think of going to buy a car without knowing what you need the car for or how much you can afford.

It is common for us to say, "I want everything done when I am sick." Often this statement is made without understanding what that could mean. It is important to comprehend the implication of "everything"—it should be based on reality. The doctors need to explain what is reasonable. They need to inform you of what is feasible and likely to help you. As described below, you will need to get the full information from your doctor. Physician Timothy Quill and his colleagues discuss this in an article in the *Annals of Internal Medicine*.[6] The phrase "Do everything" is often assumed to mean "Perform every *treatment* that focuses on controlling the disease." It is commonly forgotten that *caring* for the patient is just as important. You must give this due consideration and make an informed decision based on your own goals and values.

There are three components to the process of clarifying what is important to you and what you can do to make the process easier and to allow you to have some degree of control. The three components are as follows: (a) planning and discussing how you would like to deal with your illness, (b) appointing a surrogate decision-maker and (c) getting satisfactory information from your doctor.

PLANNING AND DISCUSSING HOW YOU WOULD LIKE TO DEAL WITH YOUR ILLNESS

For most medical situations we deal with, the discussion of what treatment to perform is easy, and most people will agree on it. If you are generally healthy and have a broken bone or obstruction of the bowel, you would like the doctors to do the best they can to fix the problem, because the chances of a favorable outcome are good.

Just talking to your loved ones about treatment preferences for even relatively simple conditions such as this opens the door to further discussion of more complex issues. If you talk about the straightforward problems with your family, the discussion may move on naturally to consideration of more difficult problems. Your spouse may ask, "But if things don't go well, what should we do?" That will open your mind and the minds of your loved ones to think more deeply. Not only will your own values be discussed, but your family may start considering how they themselves would like to be treated. It may lead to a discussion of, at least, the broad principles that would guide your plans and those of your loved ones. Ignoring and avoiding such planning could cause problems if there is a sudden illness.

One of the consequences of avoiding conversations about sickness and death is that at the time of crisis, decisions get made in a panic without consideration of all aspects of the illness. These may be decisions that you will regret later. Many people do not think about what is important to them. If they think about it, they do not talk to anyone about it. They do not talk to their family members, their friends or their doctors. Such a conversation is difficult but reduces the chances of greater difficulties when you get seriously sick.

To be helpful, the conversation should include issues like:

Do I want to do all that medical science has to offer, or do I want only treatments that have a reasonable chance of helping me?

If I lose my capacity to make my own decisions, who should make them on my behalf (someone whom you trust, who shares your values and who will be available)?

At the time of critical illness, do I want to be placed in an intensive care unit (ICU), and if my heart were to stop, do I want CPR?

It is not possible, nor is it necessary, for you to spell out all the details. There are many variables, and new decisions that have to be made every time there is a change. Just having a broad conversation to give you a general sense of what you feel makes a big difference. If you have given your family, friends and doctors a general sense of what you would like to be done, you will have helped your family, your friends, your doctors and ultimately yourself.

An unfortunate reality has recently come to light. Some doctors have been found to be ignoring some patients' advance directives—perhaps because of a misunderstanding of the directives or a misunderstanding of the law. But such disregard of the patient's wishes also occurs because some doctors have a different perspective from that of the patient and family, and they willfully ignore the directives. The law is clear that doctors must follow the advance directives, and charges have been filed in some cases where doctors did not comply.[7]

One example cited was the case of Bucilla Stephenson, who was 91 and terminally ill. In March 2012, clinicians at Doctors Hospital of Augusta installed a breathing tube in her throat and placed her on mechanical ventilation. This was contrary to Stephenson's advance directive and contrary to the specific directions of her designated health-care agent (her granddaughter).[8]

To help protect yourself from similar violations of your wishes, once you have had the discussion and have thought about your goals and what you would like, it would be helpful if you wrote these thoughts down on paper with your name and the date. Even stating that you had the discussion and the broad decisions you made will be helpful to your family and to your doctors, as well. Also, encourage your family members to do the same. It should be your (and their) own decision made freely, without pressure from anyone. Making your wishes known in writing helps everyone involved. Furthermore, if you change your mind, you can make your new wishes clear at any time—just document, sign and date the changes.

In *Knocking on Heaven's Door*, Katy Butler offered the simple and useful suggestion of writing a "legacy letter" to one's family and friends. It can be framed in any way you want. Inspired by her, I wrote the following legacy letter to my son and daughter-in-law:

July 17, 2014

Dear Saurabh and Cary,

I was at a book reading of Knocking on Heaven's Door *by Katy Butler. She suggested that writing a "legacy letter" was a good way to communicate one's thoughts, desires and wishes to the family.*

We have discussed this before, and I have it in my will that I would like to have comfort and peace and my family and friends around me during the time before death. Obviously no one has any idea how and when I will die, but prolonging the dying process is something I do not want.

I do not want to go to a Nursing Home or Assisted Living facility. I would rather hasten my death than be dependent in that kind of facility.

If I have a disability (difficulty walking or use of limbs or speech problems) and I have adequate mental capacity, I will make my decisions. But if I cannot, I do not want to be just dragged along.

If I lose my mental capacity, I do not want to be given food and water if I cannot take it myself. Give access to food and water but do not feed me. That is a legal and a simple way to hasten my death in that situation.

With regard to the disposal of my body, I would like it to be used for medical science and for other people as appropriate. I have written to a friend who works in the Office of the Medical Investigator to provide information on the logistics.

I have had a good life and do so now. I am comfortable in a material sense, have an interesting life and lots of friends. I am able to keep a good relationship with you guys and the kids and I hope I remain healthy for some more time. I hope the illness before death is short.

It does feel good to have written this letter. I think Katy Butler's suggestion was a good one and will suggest it to my readers.

Remember, talking about sex does not make you pregnant and talking about death does not kill you.

Pops

Such a letter can serve as a conversation-starter and will help you as well in writing down your wishes for your physicians. It is not easy, but you will have a sense of relief and freedom if you can do it. Such a discussion is also considered an advance directive. There are many versions of this, but the key is to let your wishes be known to your family, your friends and your doctors.

APPOINTING A DECISION-MAKER

It is also helpful and advisable that you appoint someone you trust to be your spokesperson for matters related to your health in case you are unable to speak for yourself. If you do get sick, you or your surrogate will need input from your doctors in order to make decisions about the disease and how you would like it to be treated. To make decisions about a specific illness, you need to consider your condition and the status of your general health at that time. You might make different decisions if you are weak and old than if you are young and generally healthy.

The decision-maker should be someone you trust and someone who knows you and your values. This may or may not be your next of kin. For example, you may not want to burden your husband with this role if he is in frail health himself, and you would not want to appoint a daughter who lives in a distant state and would not be able to be at your bedside promptly. The decision-maker, your spokesperson, can speak for you and decide for you if you are not able to. That is why your discussion with all those close to you is necessary, and the decision-maker should be a part of it. The decision-maker appointed by you in writing has legal authority. These appointees are also called "proxy health care decision-makers."

GETTING SATISFACTORY INFORMATION FROM YOUR DOCTOR

When you are sick, you will go through a number of steps in which the doctors collect information about you: what you tell them (your history); what they find from examining you (physical examination results); and the tests they conduct (laboratory and imaging—X-rays and scans). This may be a simple process or a difficult and complicated one. Whatever the tests and procedures may be, your doctor should keep you informed along the way. Based on your history, the physical examination and all the tests, your doctor will be able to tell you what she knows—to whatever degree of certainty she can. Then your physician will also be in a position to discuss with you what *needs* to be done and what *can* be done.

Some doctors are good communicators, while others are not so good. Some explain the whole situation in detail in a language that is clear, without the use of technical terms. Others offer little detail and do not give clear answers that can be understood by non-medical people. The point to remember is that it is *your* life. You are entitled to full details, and you should make every effort to get a complete understanding of your situation.

Here are some pieces of information you should make every effort to get:

i. The Providers
— Name, type of training and field they work in
— Names, training and field of work of all medical personnel involved in your care and treatment
— Contact information, including method of contacting them after hours

ii. The Disease
— Name of the disease (diagnosis)
— Which parts of your body are affected
— Whether the disease is mild, moderate or severe
— Whether it is early or advanced
— Whether the rest of your body is healthy
— Whether the disease can be cured
— What would happen if no treatment were taken

iii. The Treatment
— Whether there is a treatment available
— How effective the treatment is
— How the treatment would help you
— How often the treatment works
— The chances of the treatment helping you in particular
— If the treatment is effective, how long the benefit can be expected to last
— How long you will need to take the treatment

— The side effects of the treatment

— The cost of the treatment

— Whether, if the treatment does not work, there are other treatments available

These are broad suggestions designed to get you the basic information about your disease and what to expect. The format, even though it is an outline, provides a framework for you. Each of these simple questions and the answers to them will likely generate more questions. Do not hesitate to ask further questions, and do not hesitate to ask for an explanation of anything you do not fully understand. The doctor should be able and willing to answer all of your questions. There is a general saying that a good doctor will answer all of the questions to *your* satisfaction, though some answers may not be what you want to hear. That is your right—to be informed—and you must exercise it. It is helpful to have a trusted friend or family member with you when talking to your doctor. Taking notes and recording the conversation also can be of great help.

Like any group of people, not all doctors are the same. Some are more open than others. The reason for their hesitation to have an open discussion could be just their nature, but it may also be related to their difficulty in giving bad news. The point to remember is that it is your body, and you should exercise your right to be fully informed. We should accept that we cannot always understand all the details and fine points of all the things we deal with in our lives. Being fully informed does not mean that as a patient you will know all that the doctor knows. You don't need to, but you should understand what applies to you.

Knowledge of health-related technical terms and their meaning is often referred to as "health literacy." This varies from person to person depending on previous exposure to medical situations. The point is that the doctor must explain the situation in a language that the patient and family comprehend. If he uses terms that are not clear to you, it is appropriate, indeed necessary, that you ask him to explain them. If you or a member of the family has difficulty understanding or expressing yourselves in English, request that the physician translate into a language you are comfortable with or that your medical team provide a translator. Ask for time to understand the information given to you. Ask for more clarification if you need it. It is in your best interest to make your decision when and only when you feel that you have adequate information. It is important that you feel empowered by the information you get. Ask as many questions as it takes for you to feel that you can make an informed decision about your treatment and your life. Do not allow yourself to become a victim of an "information gap."

Some doctors may be dismissive or evasive about the information they give you. Do not accept that. Feel satisfied that you understand what it means to have the disease, the tests and the treatments. Another approach is to ask to speak to other patients in similar situations or to meet with another doctor (in other words, ask for a second opinion).

After obtaining and understanding the information, it is helpful to set your goals for your treatment and care—goals that are realistic but may need to be modified as time passes.

Planning is always important, but here we will discuss planning regarding major illnesses that will drastically change your life or where there is a high chance of your dying from them. The situations and diseases of this type, to name just a few, include progressive and degenerative neurological problems (large stroke, progressive dementia, Lou Gehrig's disease), severe heart failure or myocardial infarction (heart attack), kidney failure, lung damage (e.g., emphysema), joint damage (arthritis) and certain forms of cancer. Severe traumas including major burns and motor vehicle injuries also fall into this category.

The number and types of illnesses and problems listed above are varied, as are patients; each situation is different and needs to be looked at on an individual basis. Added to this complexity is the patient's health and functional status before the current illness or accident occurred. For this reason, only general guidelines can be given. The main point is worth repeating—you and your family must be fully informed about the good and the bad, and decisions need to be made jointly between the doctor and you or, if you are unable to do so, the person you designated in advance. Clear understanding of the treatments is vital, including how often and to what degree a given treatment works and the problems that may arise from it. These questions may sound simple, but they must be answered to your satisfaction.

When a person is faced with fatal or life-altering illness, two major psychological responses occur. The first could be called a "numb" feeling. Many patients and family members are so severely surprised and affected by the news that they are unable to think properly. Even if capable of making difficult decisions in their day-to-day lives, they become quiet, unable to think clearly and unable to analyze the situation; they become dependent on others to guide them. Some people call this "shock." I met a gentleman who was an accomplished engineer who could not find his driver's license and Social Security card in his wallet. He just put his wallet on the table, and his friends had to take them out. His wife had died in a car wreck, and his two children were in the ICU. Gradually, over the next few days, he recovered his normal capacity—both the children survived with minimal damage. Such instances of emotional shock are common and may be called normal under the circumstances.

The other common response is that of denial, discussed in chapter 1. Denial is a major issue during serious illness or when facing death. Denial is a normal response to physical and emotional trauma; its intensity varies, it manifests itself in different ways, but it is real. Denial means that the patient does not accept that he or she has a serious illness, all evidence to the contrary.

It is the responsibility of the doctors and the medical team to work with your or your family member's denial and overall emotional state so that you the patient do not suffer further hurt. Denial can lead to decisions that are not in your best interest. It is the responsibility of the physicians and other health-care providers and members of the patient's circle to deal with this distressing reality by interacting with the family in a kind and sensitive manner. The "denial response" to tragedy can last for varying periods of time. The actual duration depends on the specific circumstance. During the period of denial by the patient or the family, it is up to the medical providers to help them all deal with the situation in a way that leads to the patient having the best outcome possible under the circumstances. There is another tool that is helpful but not used often enough: if the doctor asks the patient to repeat what he heard in his own words, it helps the patient think more realistically.

Communication among different family members is also very important. The patient's family members should talk to each other and express their hopes, goals and doubts. This is not easy, but it is helpful. Assistance is sometimes available through family and friends who are trusted by you but are not emotionally devastated and are still able to understand the gravity and reality of your situation, both medical and emotional. This liaison can ask the questions you are unable to ask. Such a person can act as a link between the doctors and you. If the doctors want to talk openly—giving grave news and discussing options—this person can help to foster a dialogue. If the medical providers are hesitant or unable to initiate the conversation, this person can persuade the doctors and nurses to arrange meetings between the two groups. Such conversations may need to occur on several occasions, as appropriate to the situation.

Interestingly, there is another phenomenon, "provider denial," that may interfere with a realistic assessment of the situation. Some doctors are so focused on being positive and optimistic that they deny the medical reality—not just to the patient but even to themselves. Some psychologists have stated that denial is a form of self-delusion. The doctors, somehow, convince themselves that all will be well despite what the facts indicate. The doctors persuade themselves that the treatment they have in mind will cure the patient or at least fix the problem. They give an overly optimistic picture to the patient that makes the patient feel good in the short term. This has been called "the tyranny of the positive." You may make plans based on the optimism of the doctor and then be hurt when reality sets in; your hopes are dashed when the situation worsens, causing damage at both a psychological and a physical level.

If the two responses of numbness and denial are not too severe, the patient and family may be able to get the providers to answer the questions outlined above. The responsibility of holding such conversations does lie with the doctors. Unfortunately, too often they do not follow through, and you are the one who suffers because of poor understanding of the reality or because unnecessary procedures and treatments may be performed on you.

To summarize: patients and families must take upon themselves the task of getting complete and accurate information about the illness and treatment options before making a decision. They must make *informed* decisions. After due deliberation and information-gathering, if you decide that the treatment suggested to you by your medical team is right for you, you should go ahead with it. Otherwise, you should decline. In either case, you have a right to delay your decision until you are satisfied that you have the information you need in order to make it.

Remember, we are not discussing standard, effective treatments in this context. We are discussing treatments for patients for whom previous treatments did not work or for whom the disease returned after an initial period of success. We are looking also at patients who have multiple medical problems in whom treatment of one disease may be detrimental to the other. Further, patients who are elderly with chronic debility may not tolerate some treatments.

In such individuals, the body is in a delicate state of balance with little reserve. Even minor stress (like hernia surgery) can cause major complications. When dealing with such a situation, decisions have to be thought out and made with especially careful deliberation.

If you have doubts about taking a suggested treatment or if you feel the doctors are withholding a treatment that could benefit you, you have the option of asking for a second opinion or requesting help from the hospital's ethics committee. If you feel that the doctors are pushing you toward taking a treatment about which you have doubts, ask for a second opinion. Do the same if you feel that you are being denied a treatment that would help you. This will provide you with the opportunity to discuss your questions and misgivings with a physician who has a different perspective. If the second doctor also says that a treatment that you requested is not suitable for you, her opinion may help you to accept the reality and understand the reasons why the first doctor does not want to give you the treatment. On many occasions I have referred patients for a second opinion if I felt uncertain. There were situations where I thought the treatment was not in the patient's best interest, but I wanted to be sure.

Seeking a second opinion also will give you more time to think and reflect on the issues, and it may clarify any doubts that arose during your previous discussions.

Additionally, all hospitals have ethics committees whose main role is to improve communication between the medical teams and the patient. Such third-party interventions are very useful. The ethics committee is helpful in resolving disagreements. If you and your doctors disagree, the committee adds to the communication. They have you and your doctors express why each party wants or does not want a particular treatment. Such a dialogue in the presence of a third party opens up channels of communication.

If you consent to a treatment about which you may have had misgivings, you can see how the situation evolves—what course the illness takes and what benefits and problems the treatment results in. After a trial, you can change your mind; you can ask for the treatment to be stopped. This is a step-by-step process, and the situation can and should be re-evaluated as needed.

If you decide not to take further active treatment, you have many options— options that are focused on comfort, relief of symptoms and quality of life. There are many facilities, organizations and specialists whose goal is your comfort. The approach they use is a combination of symptom control, social support and help with logistics. They can work with you whether you are at home or in a nursing home or similar facility. The medical providers in this system have special training in controlling your symptoms. They know how to help with pain and shortness of breath, the two most common problems with terminal illness. They can also help in making adjustments for trouble with mobility, eating and water intake. They can provide help with issues related to bladder and bowel function. In some cases, medical interventions are needed to relieve certain symptoms. For example, fluid buildup around the lung or in the abdomen may require drainage in a hospital; your comfort team can help with that too. Even when you are under "comfort care," you can go to the hospital for such acute problems.

At a logistical level, these organizations and specialists can assist with facilities or devices to make life easier for the patient, like special beds, bed-side commodes and chairs that make it easier to shower. They help with obtaining medications and doctor visits if needed. They function as a team and work together to provide you with comfort in a variety of ways. If you need spiritual counseling, that is also available.

At the time of death, they help keep the patient comfortable and at peace. They even assist the family after death with the multiple tasks that need to be done.

A number of groups come under the broad umbrella of comfort care, hospice and palliative care specialists being the two most common. Under each, there are many people with specific training, all working toward the goals of your comfort and easing the burden on you and your family. Details of how you can take advantage of these facilities can be obtained from your doctor, nurse or social worker. You can also get more information from Katy Butler's excellent book, *Knocking on Heaven's Door*.[9] On page 288 she gives a comprehensive list of comfort care sources. After dealing with the difficulties of her father's last illness, she compiled this resource guide to help everyone in similar situations.

Compassion and Choices is an organization that provides information on health-care planning. They are a resource for Advance Care Planning, for comfort care, and, if desired, for information on hastening one's death when terminally ill. They can be reached at 1-800-247-7421 or CompassionAndChoices. org.

The option of comfort rather than active treatment of an advanced, untreatable disease should not be viewed as a "last resort" or as an "act of desperation." Comfort should be looked upon as a new approach to management of the patient as a person who has a change of goal. A goal toward comfort before death. This is discussed in more detail in chapter 13.

6

Do No Harm

"First, do no harm." It is a common adage in medicine, said to have been initially verbalized by Hippocrates, the Greek physician from the fifth century before the Common Era (BCE).[1] It has usually been interpreted to mean that the physician should not do anything that may hasten the patient's death. Putting it in the perspective of its long history requires understanding what was available to physicians at different times. Before the twentieth century, there was no treatment for infectious disease, and surgery was limited to amputation of injured or damaged limbs. Surgery of more complex nature was only possible after the availability of anesthesia in the late nineteenth century. Based on their misunderstanding of the causes of disease, bloodletting was practiced by many physicians before modern times. Other available and still accepted treatments, such as opiates for pain, alleviated symptoms, but they did not control the underlying problem.

As the understanding of diseases improved, doctors stopped utilizing many treatments that were causing more harm than good, and the injunction "First, do no harm" became important again. This was a useful and helpful approach toward patients. In the early days, supporting patients until they recovered on their own was the best that physicians could do. In that context, the old adage was a good approach to medical treatments. As medical science progressed, as more effective treatments became available and more could be done to cure patients or enable them to live with chronic diseases, "First, do no harm" remained a useful guide for trying to help patients recover. During these attempts to improve treatments, some patients admittedly were harmed, but through systematic use of new ways of treating many diseases, countless other patients have been helped.

In our current age, the rate of improvement has slowed down. The law of diminishing returns is in effect, as it inevitably will continue to be. The first decades of the twentieth century saw clean water and safe food, the development of antibiotics and insulin, and other advances in public health and medical science. We are now faced with a different problem. Even though many patients are helped, many others receive only partial benefit. Some manifestations and effects of the disease are controlled, life may be prolonged, but pain or other problems are not reduced. The meaning of "Do no harm" has been doctored again. Obviously, dying prematurely from an illness is a harm. But some feel that prolongation of a painful life is also a harm. This is one of the most difficult and contentious issues in medicine and medical ethics today; the issue is one with no clear answers and one where limits cannot be defined.

One issue worth discussing, however, is this: Is pain a harm? Many would agree that it is. The next question is: How should it be dealt with? What approaches are possible and worth considering? It is important to clarify that, as explained in the preface, "pain" (as I use the word in this book) is a broad term. It includes not just physical agony but also many symptoms and manifestations that are distressing or limit the patient's capability of carrying on a reasonable life—a life that is satisfying to her. The medical approach to pain, in its broadest meaning, is manifold. The first step, obviously, is to remove the source of pain or control it with whatever means are reasonable and available.

One important question that society, its leaders and the medical professionals should ask is: If the treatment available for a given disease, in a given patient, provides only partial benefit with a high chance of a painful subsequent existence, should it be undertaken? There are many ramifications to this question, and it is safe to say there is no answer that will feel satisfactory to everyone. However, just raising the issue at an individual and societal level will help reduce frustration and hardship. It is common for patients and medical professionals to undertake treatments just because they are available. Doctors often give treatments because "they are there" without thinking of their multiple consequences. This one simple step of thinking of the risks and benefits, short term and long term, will lead to wiser decision-making and is likely to reduce some of the pain mentioned above. On an individual level, the decision needs to be made between the patient and physician. But thinking about the question by both separately will lead to more reasonable decisions.

"Don't play God" is a common phrase in day-to-day life. In medicine it is used regularly in the context of a dying patient. Interestingly, it is employed almost exclusively when a doctor says that the time has come to stop treatments that have not helped the patient; all known, reasonable treatments have been tried, without benefit, and the current treatment has not achieved the basic goal of controlling the disease or reversing its effects. In these situations, some physicians will suggest that the treatment be stopped and all available means to keep the patient comfortable be utilized until death comes, as it will. At such times family members may accuse the doctor of playing God, implying that the physician is condemning the patient to death. They insist that it is only God's prerogative to say when a person dies. Stopping treatment is not for the doctor to decide, they say; only God can decide. Some even say that God will make a miracle happen. The patient will recover. They say that the doctor should follow God's will and continue treatments. Such an accusation is obviously disconcerting. No reasonable doctor wants to take over God's role.

Those who say that the doctor is playing God by withholding or withdrawing a treatment aimed at controlling the disease disregard the obvious medical facts. They lose sight of the reality that the patient's disease has not responded to previous medical attempts to treat it. For unclear reasons, they feel that treatments must be continued until death actually occurs. In their minds ceasing active treatments is playing God.

Let us look at the situation from another perspective. If a patient has an advanced stage disease for which there is no known potentially effective treatment, accepting that reality is a reasonable response. In such cases, accepting reality means ceasing treatment. What about the doctor who tries to treat a patient in that setting, ignoring all known experience and acting irrationally based on an unclear thought process? The doctor who tries to treat a patient when there is no chance of benefit is actually the one "playing God." Going against knowledge, experience and medical reality is playing God.

It is interesting that the doctor who follows the evidence and takes the facts into account is the one more likely to be accused of playing God. The doctor who rejects the evidence and ignores the facts is lauded because she did not give up. Presumably, this irrational thinking is a reflection of the attitude, prevalent in many of us, that we must try everything even though the "everything" is vague and is known to cause pain and other distress.

Treatments undertaken without consideration of the pros and cons can cause harm and consequent regrets—and may be futile as well. They may have some effect, but it may not be enough to offset the harm. The treatment may cause anxiety and stress to health-care providers and waste the resources of society. If a decision is made after due deliberation, a poor outcome is easier to accept. Let us not resort to the modern version of bloodletting. President George Washington was subjected to many bloodlettings that may have hastened his death. Let us weigh our decisions to avoid predictable harm.[2]

At a societal level, a vigorous thinking, re-thinking and debate are due. The questions to consider include "Are we causing harm in the pursuit of doing good?" "Should there be limits?" "Should there be more consideration given to secondary effects of what appears to be progress?" These are big questions. But the debate has started, led by, among others, bioethicist Daniel Callahan, one of the pioneers at the medical ethics institute, the Hastings Center. He says we should think carefully about the good *and* the bad that come from any treatment.[3]

The best way to avoid harm from unproven treatments, or from treatments that are not likely to help, is to think about the benefits and risks that a given treatment will bring. Thinking and analyzing rather than jumping into an action can protect many patients from harm. Actions cause more harm than thought does.

As discussed above, pain in any form is a harm to the patient. We should do our best to eliminate or reduce it. In the ideal situation, this can be achieved by controlling the disease that is causing the pain. However, in some cases, the disease cannot be controlled. For those cases, there are methods of relieving the painful symptoms even without controlling the disease. In rare instances, controlling patients' pain is not possible despite all available methods and drugs. In such cases, a radical approach to control pain is gaining momentum around the country. This approach has been advocated for patients who are expected to die from their disease in the near future and for whom it has become clear that there is no way that the progression of the disease can be stopped. If a patient is in pain (physical or other) and the *patient* feels that the pain is causing harm, another alternative is available. That is the use of the Physician Aid in Dying (discussed in detail in chapter 13). If the pain is causing harm, harm enough that the patients want relief by hastening their own deaths, medical help achieving this end should be permissible and legal, as it is in California, Oregon, Washington, Montana and Vermont.[4] In such cases assisting patients to hasten their own deaths (by providing them with prescriptions to end their own lives at a time of their choosing) is not a harm. Because the pain is the harm, aiding patients in this manner is not harming them.

7

Statistics
They Help and They Fool

There is the old joke that there are lies, damn lies and statistics. It is unfortunately true that some people with an agenda use statistics to fool other people. By selective presentation, by misusing statistical methods, they can convince others of the validity of a statement they want to make. Those maneuvers may be officially sanctioned and valid but can be deceptive. It takes a lot of effort to understand the *real* meaning and significance of the information.

It is common practice in clinical trials to show that a new drug is better than the old drug. That is the basis of approval of the new drug by the Food and Drug Administration (FDA). Suppose the old drug reduces the blood pressure by an average 10 mm and the new drug reduces the blood pressure by 12 mm. In terms of the health of the patient and how the patient feels, this makes no difference. However, by looking at the data in different ways and analyzing it by multiple methods, it often is possible to show a "statistically significant" improvement with the new drug compared to the old one. With that, new, expensive and profitable drugs get approval.

Of course, no one can beat the advertising industry when it comes to misusing statistics for personal gain. Statistics can be employed to make a point even if it really makes no meaningful difference. Advertisers use numbers to sell their product. They use phrases like "25 percent better" without explaining "Better than what?"

On the other hand, proper and honest use of statistics can distinguish between coincidence and a real relationship between two events. It was through rigorous statistical analysis that it could be proven that cigarette smoking causes lung cancer and throat cancer. Not every smoker develops lung cancer, and some patients get lung cancer even though they never smoked. However, statistical analysis of smoking history and development of lung cancer clearly established that non-smokers get much less lung cancer and certain other diseases.

On a day-to-day basis, we find that statistical information is difficult to understand. Two examples bring out the point. The chances of winning a lottery are very small. But millions of people buy lottery tickets. Say that a one-dollar ticket gives you a *chance* to win a million dollars. That may seem worthwhile—a dollar to win a million! What is the harm? Well, if two million people buy the lottery tickets, your chances of winning go down seriously. One reason we continue to buy lottery tickets is that the one person who wins the lottery is talked about in the media, so we get hyped up. The two million who bought tickets that did not win are not talked about. The sponsor gets a million dollars out of the deal, and two million people are disappointed.

The other example comes from modes of travel. Many people are afraid to fly in an airplane but do not worry about driving to their destination. Analysis of the data has shown that commercial air travel entails much less risk of death or injury than travel by car. Yet those who are afraid of flying remain afraid. One reason is that if an airliner crashes, it makes the headlines, while car crashes are common enough that they receive little publicity. So despite clear statistics, we have our fears and prejudices, and we do what feels comfortable to us. When dealing with serious medical problems, we must understand the real meaning of the statistics we are given.

Another way that statistics are helpful is to determine risk. Risk is difficult to understand as shown by the perception of the risk of driving and flying.

In medicine, as a patient and as a medical provider, understanding statistics about risk is very important but can be quite difficult. We are regularly and frequently told of the risk of this or that food, of one or another behavior or of how a drug can reduce the risk of heart attack or kidney stones. The statements are probably truthful; they are based on information collected on individuals and groups of people. The data are accumulated and analyzed and made public. We need the information; we can benefit from it. Several problems arise to make this difficult. The first is that the amount of information we need to understand and interpret can be overwhelming. Related to that are the media. They try to simplify the information, and this ends up confusing us further by over-simplifying complex problems. Think of the number of times you have been told that blackberries or radishes or red wine are good for you. But you never find out how much benefit you get.

Studies have limitations, and most of us cannot critically evaluate the conduct of the study to look for those limitations and problems. So we have to rely on the people who designed and conducted the study to reveal its flaws. They may or may not do that, depending on how they want to use the data. If they want to get personal benefit from the results, they may not be truthful. Sometimes, the people who design and conduct the study do not recognize the problems. A simple approach for us is to get the information, think about it and apply a healthy skepticism to the conclusions and meaning of what we hear. Let us look at some real-life situations in medicine.

It is now well known that if a person has a heart attack, his chances of getting a second heart attack are greater than someone's who has never had one. By comparing the information on healthy people and patients after a heart attack, researchers could state with certainty that indeed a second heart attack was a significant risk for those who had one heart attack. The next step was to find out if that risk could be reduced. A number of patients who had had a heart attack were followed for a long period of time. Some were given no additional treatment but were tracked to determine how they fared. Another group was treated with drugs that experts thought might reduce the risk of a second heart attack. Many such clinical trials were conducted. By comparing the heart attack rates in the two groups, researchers found that certain drugs did indeed reduce the incidence of second heart attacks. Thus, after examination of the data and statistical analysis, these drugs became a part of the standard treatment after a heart attack.

Statistical science is a mathematical system that makes calculations based on available data and attempts to generalize the information to larger groups. For example, scientists study the relationship between obesity and heart disease. They take a certain number of people who are obese and a certain number of people who have normal weight. They determine the number of people in each group who have heart disease. They do not study everyone. They find that there is more heart disease in the obese population than in the non-obese group. Thus, they can, by a series of calculations, make a general statement that obesity is a risk factor for heart disease. (Gallup polls use the same method when they try to predict which candidate will win an election.) Researchers take a sample of the population and generalize from that data, a complex process. It may not be foolproof, but it provides reasonable probability.

Based on these calculations and the differences in occurrence of heart disease in these groups and sub-groups, scientists called epidemiologists try to predict what will happen to the population as a whole. The calculations become more and more complex as new parameters are studied.

In other diseases, too, such clinical trials have been performed. They produced significant results in some but not in others. The results of these trials form the basis of treatments recommended for that disease. Conducting these trials is complex. There are many variables and details. Each disease has sub-groups—for example, women who have heart disease, men under 45 who have heart disease, smokers who have heart disease—and there are many drugs that are potentially useful. Studies are ongoing, and doctors try to keep abreast of the results and adopt treatments as answers become available. However, doctors are also influenced by drug salespeople and advertising.

When informed about the results of a study, patients need to discuss the recommendations with their health-care providers and understand the benefits and risks, as discussed in chapter 5. Is the improvement small or large? Are the side effects mild or severe? Only after understanding the risks and benefits should you as the patient agree to the treatment. Unfortunately, the answers can be complicated and often not black and white. You need to think about what is in your best interest and then decide. Two Hollywood celebrities' stories bring out the complexity and difficulty of interpreting risks.

In 2001 television actress Suzanne Somers was diagnosed with stage two breast cancer.[1] After her surgery (a lumpectomy followed by radiation), she was advised to take chemotherapy to reduce the risk of her cancer returning. The risk of recurrence after treatment of the primary breast cancer could have been between 10 percent and 70 percent depending on the details of her disease, which I do not have. Somers chose not to take chemotherapy and to use instead the herbal medication Iscadon, a derivative from mistletoe claimed to strengthen the immune system, along with "positive thinking," growing her own organic vegetables, sleeping at least nine hours a night and exercising daily. She ascribed her remaining free of cancer to these actions. The point is that even in the worst case, she had about a one in three chance of not having a recurrence. It remains unclear if she would have benefited from the chemotherapy that was recommended to her, just as it remains unclear whether the path she chose was the reason for her remaining free of cancer.

What we know is that those who take chemotherapy reduce their risk of recurrence. The actual amount of reduction depends on the specific features of the cancer. This is a major problem with regard to assessment and perception of risk, a problem that cancer specialists and cancer patients face frequently. There is no sure answer either way. The success of Somers' books demonstrates the desire of many individuals to exercise some control over their cancer and its possible recurrence.

The other celebrity example is Angelina Jolie, who underwent a double mastectomy in 2013 without having ever been diagnosed with cancer of any kind.[2] In her case, her mother had developed breast cancer at an early age, and her grandmother and an aunt both had died of cancer. Jolie discovered that she had a mutated form of the BRCA1 gene, which she was told was associated with an 87 percent chance of her developing breast cancer and a 50 percent chance of her developing ovarian cancer during her lifetime. The numbers can be looked at in many ways. She chose to have a double mastectomy, which would reduce the chances of breast cancer to low levels; two years later she followed up with removal of her ovaries and fallopian tubes. Based on her analysis of the risk of cancer, she chose to have the surgeries. This was her decision based on her perception of risk and benefit.

In our day-to-day lives, we face the question of certainty. We make some assumptions, and they serve us well. A common situation is when we talk to a friend and say, "I will see you at four o' clock tomorrow." The chances of being able to get to the appointed place at the appointed time are very good—you feel certain that you will be there. But think what may happen—note I said "may," not "can"—between now and four o' clock tomorrow. Something could come up at work that you have to deal with; your car might not start, there could be a traffic jam, and so on. Further, you could get sick, or you could be the victim of a drive-by shooting. The point is that one cannot be *absolutely* certain. We make our decisions based on the understanding that those events that could prevent you from meeting your friend happen so infrequently that they can be ignored.

Similar issues of certainty and uncertainty come up when dealing with medical decisions. The use of another vague but useful concept is that of "reasonable." We use it in our lives regularly as described above. We need to use that concept in medicine; otherwise, we can cause harm by doing too much or not doing enough. When looking at simple problems, we can say we are certain about some things. A child breaks a bone by falling off a bicycle. Can we say with absolute certainty that the bone will heal if the break is given proper treatment? No, not really. A number of things have been known to go wrong. But we can say with *reasonable* certainty that the bone will heal normally.

Taking "certainty" to the other end of the difficulty spectrum, we can think of an 85-year-old who has been a lifelong smoker and has been house-bound on oxygen for many years. He has a stroke that paralyzes one-half of his body. Can we be certain that he will need oxygen for the rest of his life? Yes. Can we be certain that he will die in the next 20 years? Yes. Can we be certain that he will recover sufficiently to leave the hospital? No.

If over the next few days, the patient's kidneys start failing and his lungs fill up with fluid and it takes more and more effort to get enough oxygen to his body, will he recover? Can we be certain that he will not recover? Some physicians will say they are certain he will *not* recover. Others might say they are reasonably certain that he will not recover. If over the following day or so his lung function and his kidney function get worse, most physicians will say they are certain he will not recover. The point is that because the difference between reasonable certainty and absolute certainty depends on a number of factors that are changeable, the distinction is not clear-cut.

When dealing with such situations, the patient, the family and the doctors need to look at all the parameters involved in the patient's condition and make decisions after considering the whole picture. Reasonable certainty in most situations should guide us. If we only work with absolute certainty, we are more likely to hurt patients than help them. Similarly, would we treat the broken bone of a child even though there is no *absolute* certainty the bone will heal? Of course, we would.

Our decisions in life in general and in medical situations need to be based on reasonable certainty and not on absolute certainty. Even our criminal justice system is based on reasonable certainty—hence the phrase "beyond a reasonable doubt."

We need to guide our lives and our response to illness on the principle of *reasonable* certainty.

The statistician's role is to determine what information is real and what is not. Statisticians make assumptions and calculations, and they work with other experts to decide what to study and to what degree difference between the two groups of participants is meaningful. Since they are studying only a small part of the population, they need parameters to decide what is important and what is not. A common benchmark is to determine *statistical* significance. Statisticians cannot determine what is important and what is relevant for the medical problem under study. They can only determine the statistics and calculate how "real" the difference is between the two groups. Determination of *statistical* significance is their main tool. They try, by these calculations, to eliminate the element of chance. Statistical significance is only one parameter, albeit an important one. The researcher working with patients or studying a particular disease needs to determine whether the differences are meaningful and important. They need to go beyond just the statistical significance.

As an example, suppose that a major pharmaceutical company advertised its newly released drug for high blood pressure. Running in all the major medical journals aimed at cardiologists and general internists, the ad featured a graph that showed that the new drug offered "30 percent better control" over the available generic. Such a graph would look impressive, until you examined it closely. Suppose that the cheap generic drug leads to 92 percent control of blood pressure and the new expensive drug gives 95 percent control. That small difference would not make the patient feel any better and would not significantly lower his risk of heart attack or stroke.

The researcher has to determine if the differences are *meaningful and important*. Using the data and basing recommendations on it is the responsibility of the researchers doing the study. This should be explained to the patient fully and clearly. But the patient also has a responsibility to ask relevant questions and become informed. In his 2011 book *Your Medical Mind*, Jerome Groopman describes a woman who did this.[3] She had mildly elevated cholesterol. Her doctor told her that by using a particular cholesterol-lowering drug she could reduce the risk of a heart attack by 30 percent. She did further research and found that her risk of having a heart attack without the drug was about 1 percent. Thus the risk was low to begin with, and a 30 percent reduction would take it from 1.0 percent to 0.7 percent. Yes, that would constitute a 30 percent reduction, but to the patient this was not meaningful, and there would be side effects from the medication. She chose not to take it. She made an informed decision after gathering facts and analyzing them.

Statistics have quirks and can be confusing. When you hear the weatherman say, "There is a 10 percent chance of rain today," how do you react? What do you think? Some people laugh at the weatherman because it is raining at their house. What a fool he is—there is a 100 percent chance of rain at my house! Statistics can be fun. They are useful, but they can be tricky.

The point of the above is that statistics is an important field. It has helped resolve or at least improve understanding of many complex problems. But when a health-care provider gives you "statistics" about your disease or the treatment, you should ask for a more detailed explanation of what you are being told. The numbers can be looked at in many ways, and you need to have a good understanding of their meaning for you. Some doctors confuse or over-interpret the statistics. A colleague of mine once told me that a particular patient was unusual because he had lived longer than average. The reality is that half of all patients will live longer than average—that is what an average is.

Another oncologist I worked with closely was a firm believer in chemotherapy treatment of breast cancer, to reduce the risk of the cancer recurring. We had a patient with breast cancer who was calculated to have a 30 percent chance of the cancer coming back over the next five years or so. I recommended chemotherapy to reduce the chances of recurrence. For her own reasons, the patient decided not to take the treatment. Following the principle of autonomy, I agreed to withhold chemotherapy. I felt the patient had made an informed decision. When my friend heard about this he was upset. He said to me, "You know she *will* have a recurrence." The reality was that there was a 70 percent chance that her cancer would not come back. Yes, a 30 percent risk of recurrence is pretty high, but by no means can one say that she *will* have a recurrence. Some doctors use statistics to generate fear and push treatments on patients.

How does the doctor taking care of you use statistics? This varies. Sometimes it is like calling a glass half empty or half full. She reads the reports stating that a drug was effective in one-third of patients with a disease similar to yours. But similar is not the same. In fact, no two patients are the same. Doctors use their experience, knowledge and judgment to see how well the report they read fits your situation. Furthermore, their own values may influence their thinking;

so statistics are also affected by those who interpret them. When making recommendations to you, the doctors are using more than just the numbers. That can be confusing. As a patient, you should try to get as much detail as possible and make your decisions after giving full consideration to all factors, as the examples above show. Evaluating and thinking about all issues are very helpful.

Another aspect to consider is the difference between the effect and the benefit. After a new drug is tested, it may be found that the patients treated with the new drug had a significant improvement in their heart function. This is good news. However, the next equally important question is: Did the patient feel better, or did he or she live longer with a better quality of life? This is often not discussed. The point is that statistics help guide the doctors. You have to decide if what they propose will benefit you—in your particular situation, given your particular goals and values. That is what determines whether the treatment is worth trying.

Why Doctors Over-Treat
Training and Mind-Set

Even though it can be difficult to decide whether a treatment is appropriate and when it becomes "over-treatment," it is clear that many doctors recommend or go along with treatments that are not in patients' best interest and are not going to help them. "Over-treatment" here refers to unnecessary tests, as well as to excessive medications and procedures.

There are interrelated factors that go into over-treatment. Since there is no clear line separating appropriate treatment from over-treatment, in this chapter and the two that follow, I would like to analyze the process and reasons for over-treatment, beginning with their training and mind-set. This analysis will give you insights into the doctors' thinking and actions. Once you have this understanding, you will be able to make the decisions about your treatments that are the best for you.

One aspect of over-treatment is using treatments that are focused on the disease that the patient has. Obviously, this is important and has been the basis of medicine. The problem arises when a treatment has some effect on the disease but does not necessarily help the patient. The overall effect on the patient may get lost if the focus is on the disease. Sir William Osler, who laid the foundation of modern medicine, stated, "The good physician treats the disease; the great physician treats the patient who has the disease."[1] This distinction is discussed frequently in this book.

The patient-focused approach requires providing truthful information in a sympathetic manner, and that takes time. Unfortunately, the medical system as a whole does not reward providers for their efforts at building trust and for the time they spend talking (and listening) to the patient.

The other form of over-treatment is excessive tests and X-rays performed when there is no evidence that they will help the patient. Both these forms of over-treatment have been observed and examined, including in a study from the Dartmouth Medical School.[2] Although Medicare now compensates physicians $86 for a half-hour discussion about preferences for care in the event of serious illness, usually as part of an annual physical, the American medical system pays doctors more when they work actively on diagnosing or treating a disease. It also rewards use of technology. Laboratory tests, X-rays and surgical procedures are compensated more lucratively than the time taken to listen, console and comfort. This creates an environment that encourages acting on the disease rather than working on the patient's welfare. Once you understand and accept that doctors over-treat some patients and that they give less importance to the patients' comfort than to battling the disease, you should consider what *you* can do to reduce the burden of your own disease and treatment.

Over-treatment is an issue in day-to-day patient-provider interactions, but when dealing with life-threatening illness, the problem becomes very serious. If you like the idea of comfort, you have options. The first and foremost is that you can refuse any treatment you do not want to take. No one can force a treatment on you. Related questions that have come up include: Is it suicide to refuse a treatment? Is it murder not to give it? The answer to both is "No." Pope Pius XII declared in 1957 that good Catholics did not have to prolong their lives using *extraordinary means,* such as respirators.[3] There are many reasons why over-treatment and over-diagnosis are practiced by physicians. These are described in the pages that follow. Broadly, they are due to the patient's false hope, on the one hand, and the doctor's training and beliefs, on the other. As a generalization, most doctors feel that doing more is better.

Apart from doctors' avoidance of difficult discussions, there are factors leading to over-treatment that are ingrained through their training and what they see as the normal or usual behavior of their peers. Also, forces in society in general have an influence.

Following are some reasons why doctors initiate or continue treatments that many would consider futile or inappropriate—in other words, why physicians are inclined by their training and mind-set to engage in over-treatment:

a. Refusal to accept "failure"
b. Focus on the disease and not the patient
c. Use of treatments that have not been tested
d. Suboptimal understanding of medical "progress"
e. Guidelines that are employed without proper analysis
f. Belief in certain treatments

I have listed these reasons as separate entities. In reality, many of these factors act together and make the understanding of the situation even more difficult. The important point is that doctors more often over-treat than under-treat, and understanding that fact is in your best interest.

REFUSAL TO ACCEPT "FAILURE"

By their training, most doctors want to do as much as they can to control the disease process that is making the patient sick. As a result of this thinking, it is difficult for them to accept "failure"—or what they consider failure. Because of their mind-set, many doctors blame themselves for the lack of success. Since "failure" is not acceptable to them, they often suggest another treatment if the previous one did not produce the desired results. Even if the new treatment has a low chance of helping, it gives the physician a feeling of having dodged defeat.

However, if a disease does not respond to treatment, that lack of response is not due to a failure on the part of the doctor. If the treatment was appropriate but did not work, this probably was due to the inherent nature of the disease. That is not the doctor's fault. Of course, the problem needs to be analyzed, and the doctor should make sure that the correct treatment was given.

I know many physicians who feel personally responsible if a treatment they prescribe does not meet its goal. They chastise themselves; they blame themselves. They then try to find ways to counter the perceived failure by trying new treatments even though they understand (at least on some level) that these will not help the patient. If a doctor does not want to accept failure and wants to try another treatment, he must, at minimum, discuss the case with colleagues to determine if it is in the patient's best interest to try another treatment. If the second doctor gives the opinion that the treatment did not work because of the nature and stage of the disease, it would be reassuring to the doctor and to the patient. The first doctor would not blame himself, and the patient would be reassured that everything possible to treat the disease was done. Doctors need to accept the fact that not all treatments work.

FOCUS ON THE DISEASE AND NOT THE PATIENT

For the best overall outcome, there has to be a balance between focusing on the disease and thinking broadly about the welfare of the patient. In some situations, the focus needs to be on the disease. This is necessary when the patient is healthy except for a defined illness and, even if painful, the treatment is likely to restore her to a state of generally good health. Broken bones, bowel obstructions and acute lung infections are some of these common situations. After a period of perhaps painful treatments, the patient will most likely feel much better and recover; so here eliminating the problem is worthwhile.

On the other hand, the same logic does not apply for chronically ill patients. If an elderly person who has multiple other problems (dementia, advanced cancer, damaged lungs) develops a bowel obstruction, breaks a hip or has severe recurrent pneumonia, the doctors must think of the issue in more depth. Will the treatment of the new problem help the *patient*? Yes, the immediate problem may be fixed, but doing so would not make the patient well or even more comfortable. It may be better to provide him with comfort measures without trying to fix that new problem. This is when the goal and focus of treatment need to be changed. The patient's welfare becomes more important than the control of the disease.

Doctors have different thresholds at which they change their thinking and their emphasis. The examples and scenarios given above have a lot of variability. No lines can be drawn; no one lays down rules. The important point is that you as the patient and your doctors should discuss the whole picture and reach a joint decision after due thought. The benefit and harms should be analyzed, and decisions should be based on the total picture. Your overall welfare should be the main deciding factor. If the doctor is focused on the disease, which may be appropriate in some circumstances, then some details and clarification are needed. For example, sometimes even partial treatment of the disease may help a patient feel better.

There is a common belief among doctors that all possible options for treatment must be presented to the patient. They feel that it is for the patient to decide. I disagree. I feel that only *reasonable* options should be given to the patient. The doctor has the knowledge and experience to determine what treatments are likely to help. The patient does not have that information.

The feeling that all options should be presented is reinforced by the payment system. The payment system and criteria for reimbursement for drugs by Medicare (and most commercial insurance companies) are complex. But as a generalization, the Medicare experts look at data and recommendations from drug companies, published reports and expert panels, after which they agree to pay for the treatments. This approval of payment is not necessarily an endorsement for the drug in question but is often taken as that by many physicians, a phenomenon we will address in detail in the next chapter. A recommendation by a group leads to coverage by Medicare, and doctors, taking that as an endorsement, feel obligated to offer the treatment. Furthermore, they feel it will cost the patient or themselves "nothing," so if the patient asks for the treatment, they go along. The situation is complicated by the lack of payment for the time it would take for the doctor to explain to the patient why the use of chemotherapy, for example, would not be in the patient's interest. The payment by third party payers then becomes the reason for giving a toxic and ineffective treatment.

Our fee-for-service and reimbursement system adds to inappropriate treatments and discourages proper communication between patients and doctors.

Doctors' training and mind-set were demonstrated to me when I was working with two trainees in oncology. One had a patient with throat cancer that relapsed after a response that had lasted for six months. The other had a patient with lung cancer that had not responded to chemotherapy and was too advanced for surgery or radiation. As is the practice, the fellows (what advanced trainees are called) presented me with a summary of their patients' histories and the information about their scans—which showed that the cancers had grown larger.

I asked them what they would recommend for these patients. Both young doctors were up-to-date on their medical knowledge, and both knew of new treatments that were available for those types of cancer. In my discussion with them, I asked them what kind of *benefit* each patient could expect. This gave them a chance to reflect and think beyond new chemotherapy drugs. They acknowledged that the chances of the cancer responding to the new treatments were small, and that any response they did achieve would last only for a short time. And their patients might not feel better.

After they had a chance to reflect, I gave these oncology fellows freedom to recommend to their patients whatever they thought was the right course of action. One fellow felt it was his responsibility to give the patient information on a new treatment. To give respect to the fellow's opinion, I went along with his plan. When we went into the patient's room and the oncology fellow gave him the option of trying the new chemotherapy drug, the patient said, "Doc, I am done. Just keep me comfortable." We accepted what the patient wanted and referred him to hospice for comfort care. The point is that this young doctor felt it was his duty to inform the patient of all the available treatment options, even though the patient would not have benefited from them. I am glad the patient understood the limits of medical treatments.

The other fellow was further ahead in her training. She accepted the reality. She talked to the patient very sympathetically and explained that we did not have any good options for treating the cancer. Note, she indicated that there was an option but not a good one. (As I pointed out earlier, some disagree and say that *all* options should be presented to the patient. Based on my own knowledge and experience, I favor giving only reasonable options.) The patient was only in her fifties and did not have other significant medical problems; yet she accepted the fellow's recommendation to go for hospice without trying further chemotherapy. To clarify the point about hospice: as discussed in more detail in chapter 13, hospice is an organization that focuses on the patient's comfort, and the hospice personnel help the patient die comfortably and provide emotional and practical support to the family. They do not try to treat the disease.

Both fellows had done their research and had found a treatment written up in the journals that might shrink the tumor. However, one chose to mention it to the patient—and the patient refused because he was "done." The other fellow thought more broadly and made a recommendation for comfort care. These examples illustrate the complexity of decision-making.

If the doctor says there is a treatment for your disease, that is encouraging and hopeful, but you need more details. Starting with the meaning of "effective," you must get a clear understanding of the treatment. A treatment may be called effective because it eliminates the problem, like fixing a broken bone. But "effective" can be used in many other ways. For example, a treatment may increase the ejection fraction (a measure of the heart muscle's strength) of the heart from 25 percent to 35 percent (better but still low). It is appropriate to call the drug effective, but it is more important to know how much better the patient would feel even if the treatment did work. Similarly, it is important to know how often the treatment is effective. It may be justified to call a treatment effective if it improves the ejection fraction in, say, a quarter of patients. But the patient should be informed that, as best we know, the ejection fraction improves in one in four patients, and even that does not mean that one in four are cured or feel better for a meaningful duration of time.

The next step and the next piece of information the patient needs is how long the benefit will last. Based on previous experience, it may be possible to say that in about half the patients, the benefit lasted for more than six months, but the other half experienced the benefit for less than six months. When the patient has all this information, only then can his decision be called "informed"—that is, based on knowledge and understanding.

For a doctor to suggest using a new treatment just to avoid her own feeling of failure is not fair to you. Nor is it fair when the emphasis is on the disease rather than on you, the patient. When the focus is on the immediate problem and does not take into account what had happened to the patient's body before the current event occurred, the overall outcome is likely to be poor.

Using analogies is considered patronizing by some. On the other hand, many patients and families have limited exposure to the medical system, their understanding of the complexities of the body is piecemeal, and their emotional response prompts them to "do something." For this reason, an analogy may be helpful. If you have a fairly well-running car, even if it is old, you have good reason to keep it and take care of it. If the cooling system goes out and the mechanic finds that the other systems are working well, it is worthwhile to fix the cooling system. If, on the other hand, your car is really old, you have had problems with the electrical system, and when you go to have the cooling system fixed the mechanic finds that the transmission is about to break down, that is different. In that situation, you will at least rethink fixing just the cooling system.

For a variety of reasons, doctors end up focusing on the immediate problem and forget or ignore the patient's other problems that, for the moment, are not in the forefront. When this happens, it becomes our responsibility as patients to bring up these issues during the process of making our decisions about what should or should not be done. Otherwise, we can, as the old adage goes, win the battle but lose the war. Many last-ditch, long-shot treatments are compared to a

"Hail Mary" pass in football. This is a false analogy. A successful pass in the last seconds of the game may change the outcome, but there is no harm inflicted if it doesn't succeed. With last-ditch medical treatments, chance of benefit is minimal, and usually there are painful side effects or collateral damage.

Full information, discussion and thought must guide our decisions.

In his recent book *Being Mortal*, Atul Gawande describes his father's final illness.[4] The elder Gawande had a malignant tumor on his spinal cord which had nearly paralyzed him. Surgery and radiation therapy had not controlled the cancer.

Atul Gawande is a professor of surgery at Harvard Medical School; his father and mother were both doctors. The three met with a medical oncologist to discuss the possibility of chemotherapy to try to control the cancer which had caused severe damage to the nerves of both his upper and lower limbs. Following is Gawande's account of the meeting:

> The oncologist was now center stage, but she too lacked Benzel's ability to take in the whole picture. We missed it keenly. [Benzel was a good communicator.] She proceeded in the information mode. She laid out eight or nine chemotherapy options in about ten minutes. Average number is syllables per drug: 4.1. It was dizzying. He could take bevacizumab, carboplatin, temozolomide, thalidomide, vincristine, vinblastine or some other options I missed in my notes. She described a variety of different combinations of drugs to consider as well. The only thing she did not offer or discuss was doing nothing.[5]

She was focused on the disease. Gawande adds further,

> The pressure remains all in one direction, toward doing more, because the only mistake clinicians seem to fear is doing too little. Most have no appreciation that equally terrible mistakes are possible in the other direction—that doing too much could be no less devastating to a person's life.[6]

Diane E. Meier, a respected expert in the field of palliative medicine, wrote about a patient with lung cancer that had grown back after initial successful treatment. Treatment for the recurrence had not been successful. The oncologist wanted to try one more treatment. Meier was also involved in the care of the patient. When the two doctors talked, the oncologist acknowledged that this latest treatment was not going to help the patient. He, however, felt that he would be abandoning the patient if he did not try the treatment. Meier states, "It seems that giving more treatment was the only way the oncologist knew to express his care and commitment." But what the patient was seeking was assurance that she would be cared for when treatments stopped working. With Meier's help, the goal of treatment was changed to providing comfort before she died.[7]

These are examples of one reason why doctors do too much. By their training and mind-set, they believe that they must use all possible treatments directed toward the disease, often ignoring what effect the treatments have on the patient. This practice needs to be changed, and more emphasis needs to be directed toward the patient's welfare and comfort.

USE OF TREATMENTS THAT HAVE NOT BEEN TESTED

In the 1890s surgeon William Stewart Halsted, one of the founders of Johns Hopkins Medical School, noted that many women at Johns Hopkins Hospital were dying of breast cancer. He concluded, based on the understanding of cancer in the period, that the cancer was recurring because the surgeons of the day were not removing enough of the normal-looking tissue around the cancer. He thought that there were cancer cells in this "normal" area surrounding the visible tumor.[8] He pioneered a radical surgical procedure to remove large amounts of the surrounding tissue. All muscles of the chest wall and tissues in the region of the armpit were removed. Often the patient was left with an arm that did not function.

Here is a description by geriatrician Steven H. Miles in *The Hippocratic Oath and the Ethics of Medicine*:[9]

Case 3.1 When I was a child, an aunt became very sick. She began to miss the family gatherings. In those not-so-distant days, the word "cancer" was breathed, rather than spoken aloud. After some months, I was taken to see her in a hospital. It was a good-bye visit where "good-bye" were unspeakable words. She was thin and pale. Her face was the friendly face I knew, but it had a tautness that, years later, I would learn to recognize as a sign of chronic pain. I recall being horrified by her left arm. It was hugely swollen, wrapped in bandages, and propped up on pillows. A soft, bulbous hand protruded from the bandages. "How could a disease do that?" I wondered. Later, I learned that this swelling was caused by the Halsted operation.

My aunt had undergone a radical mastectomy. This operation attempted to cure breast cancer by removing all the sites where a cancer might have silently spread. In addition to the breast, the muscles of the chest, as well as the lymph nodes in the chest, armpit and lower neck were removed. Since the lymph ducts could no longer drain fluid from the arm through the nodes, the arm became swollen with edema.

Initial results suggested that more women were "cured" of cancer by the Halsted method than with the earlier less radical surgery that only removed the tumor. However, on further follow-up it was noted that the cure rate after radical surgery was not better than it was with less radical surgery. In the 1920s, attempts were made to stop the radical surgery. Halsted was a powerful man. His students were now seeding the major medical centers around the country, and they continued to follow the master's approach of radical surgery for another two decades. It was only in the 1950s that radical mastectomy was discontinued and less radical surgery became the norm. The results were the same as with radical surgery but with less difficulty for the patients. Unfortunately, in oncology and other fields of medicine, some treatments are still continued even after they are shown to be ineffective.

Based on a good *idea* some physicians will try new treatments, which is fine. However, in many cases, the new treatment may not turn out to be helpful—the idea did not work. If this is the case, the treatment should not be used anymore. Unfortunately, for a variety of reasons, some physicians continue utilizing a given treatment even when it has been shown not to be effective. Good ideas should be tested; that is how progress occurs. But all treatments, even standard treatments, should be continually reevaluated. Decisions should be made based on facts, not on ideas.

I was lucky to have had Maxwell M. Wintrobe as my mentor. He was a short man who always wore a bowtie, and he was utterly no-nonsense. Wintrobe was a pioneer in the field of clinical hematology. He was the person who placed the study of blood on a scientific basis, leading to the understanding of, among others, various types of anemias and the leukemias.

In 1965, while addressing the Association of American Physicians, Wintrobe stated, "There is so much to learn, so much to read, that there is little time to study new developments in depth. Among other pitfalls, there are those arising from coining of names and the propounding of hypotheses . . . too many assume that a name is the answer, that a hypothesis is a truth.

However hypotheses are useful in research, one must as energetically seek to prove their weakness as to support their validity."[10]

Jerome Groopman of Harvard Medical School has written many thoughtful books and articles on a variety of topics related to medicine. He has raised awareness among non-medical people about medicine in general and about how doctors and patients think and how they make decisions. Groopman's latest book, written with Pamela Hartzband, is *Your Medical Mind: How to Decide What Is Right for You.*[11] Most of the scenarios described in this book concern patients who are healthy but have to make decisions regarding, for example, high cholesterol, hip surgery in a runner or risk of heart irregularity. He and his co-author describe the complexity of decision-making in generally healthy people.

Groopman also includes case studies of people with serious illnesses. He describes the efforts of E. Donald Thomas, who pioneered bone marrow transplantation in humans in the 1950s and was awarded the Nobel Prize for Medicine in 1990. Bone marrow transplantation was a great idea—destroy the patient's diseased bone marrow and replace it with healthy bone marrow from another person. Unfortunately, bone marrow transplantation has many complications and side effects and has been proven to be effective in only a small number of diseases. Despite this, the procedure has many proponents, including Groopman. I feel that bone marrow transplantation, after more than 50 years, continues to be a good idea, but, like Halsted's radical mastectomy, it remains to be proven as a therapeutic advance.

One reason that bone marrow transplantation is advocated by the doctors who perform it may be because the bone marrow transplant centers are paid fully for all the services they perform and thus bring in large revenues. I once heard a lecture by one of the leaders in the field. She was a dynamic speaker and a highly placed professor at a major medical school. I expected to hear a lecture on the results of the studies that her team had performed. What I got instead was a half-hour presentation on how many transplants were being done at her center and around the country, how much the number of transplants was increasing every year and the rapid rate at which revenues were rising. There was no mention of the benefits of transplantation, no discussion of the survival of patients who received the procedure. It was a lecture on the benefits of transplants for the teams performing them. The benefits of bone marrow transplants to patients remain marginal, and even these are for a small number of diseases, but large numbers of transplants are still undertaken.

Groopman offers an important generalization and provides many thoughtful insights. He states, "The decision to stop treating a patient is one of the most agonizing in medicine. Doctors don't give up on many of the sickest patients for the sake of the few . . . who will survive catastrophic illness and return to life."[12]

Trying new ideas is good, but the idea must be tested. If successful, it should be implemented, assuming that the patient gives informed consent. If not, it should be abandoned.

SUBOPTIMAL UNDERSTANDING OF MEDICAL "PROGRESS"

Doctors regularly update their knowledge by reading medical journals, looking at the Internet and discussing problems with their peers and colleagues; it is essential for them to be current about medical advances. Lifelong learning is an important parameter by which the competence of physicians is judged. The amount of information that they have to obtain, digest and use in their practices can be overwhelming. They may only have time to read the highlights or the abstract of the journal article; this can lead to a misunderstanding of the information. In addition, some authors of journal articles overemphasize the importance of the results in their reports. By subtle statements, by underemphasizing or overemphasizing some conclusions, they may try to increase the perceived significance of their research or study. Even worse, some writers have a vested interest in showing their results in a positive light. Only if the article is read carefully does the real meaning become clear.

As a result, some doctors may undertake or recommend treatments that may not be all that beneficial. For you as the patient, the important point is to ask questions—not just to question the doctor, but to get a better understanding of all the risks and the degree of the expected benefits of the newly reported treatment. If your doctor recommends a new treatment based on a report in a journal, it is important to get details of the report. For example, is this the only report, or have the results been confirmed by other studies? Taking advantage of a new treatment may make sense, but only if the results are real and are applicable to you.

Doctors may read an article presenting information on a new treatment that suggests that it works for your disease when previous treatments were not effective. This gives the doctors hope—hope for you. But they may fail to read the details of the report and so do not realize that the treatment is not suitable for you. In their optimism and desire to help you, they may recommend a treatment that would not benefit you; it might even harm you. This phenomenon occurs in all fields of medicine when dealing with patients with a wide variety of diseases of different degrees of severity and with different underlying medical conditions. New drugs and treatments are more likely to be overused or wrongly used in this way. The drug companies advertise them in medical journals, hold symposiums (often with a nice dinner) and have drug representatives meet with the doctors. The authors of the article that supported the drug also have a vested interest—their standing at the university where they teach and conduct research may depend on their number of publications, and they may give talks around the country to present their results. The drug may be effective, but the methods described above may exaggerate its benefits and efficacy. Unless the treating doctors analyze the article or listen to the talks carefully, they could be misled into believing that the treatment has a higher degree of effectiveness and benefit than it actually does.

As stated, doctors update their knowledge about different aspects of medicine on a regular basis. They read journals and books and use a variety of tools through the Internet. Depending on their field of work, they may read publications like the *Journal of the American Medical Association* or the *New England Journal of Medicine,* which cover a variety of topics. Only recently have these journals given importance to those related to comfort before death. If a doctor has a special interest in heart disease or stroke, for example, she is likely to read the *American Journal of Cardiology* or the *American Journal of Neurology.* Such specialized journals contain relatively few articles on comfort care or hospice. Most of the articles on comfort care are published in journals for specialists in those fields, like the *Journal of Palliative Medicine.* These publications are not generally read by other physicians, not even by oncologists, cardiologists and others who often treat seriously ill patients.

Information obtained through the Internet usually emphasizes the latest developments in medicine. This includes new research findings, new drugs or new devices. The Internet "alerts" rarely cover issues of comfort or alternatives to active treatment of disease, because many of these bulletins are sponsored by drug companies or manufacturers of medical devices.

As a result of all these factors, an average physician's exposure to alternatives to active treatment of disease is limited and encourages him to do more to try to control the disease. Comfort care is not at the forefront in the perception of most doctors.

In their optimism, the doctors may accept the overly encouraging conclusions drawn by the authors of the article and may undertake treatments that are not necessarily helpful to you, the patient.

GUIDELINES THAT ARE EMPLOYED WITHOUT PROPER ANALYSIS

Medical organizations like the American Medical Association (AMA) and the American College of Physicians, as well as specialty organizations like the American College of Cardiology, regularly monitor medical reports. They also sponsor studies to evaluate treatments and outcomes. They study and report on preventive measures and treatment effectiveness. These reports are very important to all physicians, who need them and use them to provide the best medical care to their patients. There are, however, some limitations and pitfalls with these guidelines. To begin with, these are *guidelines*; they are not absolute rules. They need to be applied in a way that is appropriate for the individual patient.

The guidelines regarding certain tests should be adjusted to the patient's situation and not regarded as dictates from above. Two common examples are the use of mammograms and colonoscopies. Those who wrote the guidelines did not clarify that the tests should be done only when the risk from the cancer, if one were found, was greater than the inherent risk to the patient's overall condition. For example, if a patient is suffering from advanced emphysema (lung damage, usually from smoking), a small breast cancer will not change her prospects, which will be determined by the progress of the emphysema. Many doctors did not use their judgment and performed mammograms on patients who were suffering from other advanced diseases, so whatever the mammogram showed would not help them—an unfortunate example of reading the guidelines as absolute rules.

I have seen many patients who were subjected to mammograms but were very sick from lung or liver disease and not in a condition to have treatment for breast cancer if it were found. The worst case I have heard of was brought to my attention by the daughter of a 90-year-old woman who was receiving yearly mammograms and Pap smears (a test for early cancer of the cervix seen in young, sexually active women). Even if abnormal cells had been found, the risks of major surgery would have been far greater than those of a slow-growing cancer. This, I think, was not just a matter of misunderstanding the guidelines but also an example of a dishonest physician trying to make extra money.

A large study reported that mammograms found more early cancers but that the death rate from cancer was not reduced when compared to those women whose cancer was diagnosed by other means like a lump in the breast.[13] Thus, the whole premise of mammograms is debatable, but certainly a mammogram is not necessary for a 90-year-old woman.

A further point to note is that the major medical societies and professional organizations have revised many of their guidelines, a process that reflects their concerns for the health of the community. Doctors sometimes do not follow the revised guidelines. Beginning in the 1980s, many guidelines were issued. Over the years, various professional societies have evaluated the benefits and pitfalls of those. After extensive review of the information over several years, these groups compiled a list of tests that they found had not benefited patients. They called these lists "Choosing Wisely." Each organization chose five tests or procedures that they determined were not effective, were commonly done and were expensive. These lists were first published in 2012. Surveys of physicians a year later found that only some physicians were aware of the lists of five and very few were altering their practices accordingly—maybe because of ingrained habits. They had been doing these tests for a long time and believed that they helped their patients. Possibly some physicians continue to perform these tests because they provide additional revenues to them. Atul Gawande confirmed this in an article titled "Overkill" in the *New Yorker*.[14] He pointed out that many of these tests just cause more expense and do not help the patients.

A friend's father-in-law was enjoying life at the age of 85. For some reason, not related to any problems, he was subjected to a colonoscopy. This is a procedure that finds precancerous lesions in the colon—in other words, a preventive measure to reduce the risk of colon cancer. It helps some people who have an increased risk of cancer but is helpful only if the person has many years to live, since colon cancer takes a long time to grow. Most guidelines recommend not doing a colonoscopy after the age of 65. If you are 85, a colonoscopy is of no benefit.

During the colonoscopy, they found a lesion (a polyp) that required surgical resection. This was not cancer—just a non-cancerous "lesion." After surgery my friend's father-in-law experienced multiple complications, and he died from them.

The man had had no symptoms. The guidelines do not recommend colonoscopy after the age of 65. But, for some reason, his physicians performed one, and he died from complications of surgery to remove the precancerous lesion they discovered. It is well known that even healthy elderly people are at high risk of problems after surgery. The doctors misinterpreted the guidelines, and that led to the shortening of a happy life—a tragic example of doing too much.

Some physicians have advocated a patient-centered approach to planning care and treatment. Rather than undertaking treatments to "fix" everything that doctors find "wrong" with the patient, the advocates of this approach think how the abnormal finding on examination or on a test is affecting or will affect the patient. This has been called "slow medicine." What it means is "Think first, and act only if the abnormality will hurt the patient."

Gerontologist Dennis McCullough of Dartmouth Medical School is one of the leaders of the slow medicine movement. He states that slow medicine involves family, friends and neighbors as a team with health-care providers to improve the quality of *care* and the provision of day-to-day needs to the elderly and sick and to avoid inappropriate treatments and tests. Unfortunately, very few physicians act accordingly.[15]

Such guidelines per se are not issues that concern people with serious illnesses or those facing death. They are described here to make the point that many doctors follow their peers, leaders or people in authority. They surrender their knowledge and judgment to avoid direct responsibility for their actions. Guidelines also protect the doctor in case of a lawsuit. The doctor can say, "I was following the guidelines, so you cannot fault me." Guidelines also include a standard of care. For example, they state that an abnormality in the blood showing a defect in the kidney or high blood sugar must be recorded and treated. They often do not provide room for exception. It should be up to the treating doctors to use their judgment and to put the guidelines in the context of the patient under their care. For instance, treating a patient for mild increased blood sugar is not going to help if he has badly damaged lungs.

There is a downside to trying to fix everything that is "wrong," or maybe just "not perfect." It may not be fixable, but even if it is, trying to fix one thing may damage something else. Finding a balance between doing good and causing harm is a major part of decision-making in medicine, as it is in day-to-day life. I know of a patient who was fairly functional into her eighties. She had a fall and broke her hip. She had surgery to fix the broken bone. During routine blood exams after the surgery, one of the kidney tests showed a slight elevation. Although she had no discomfort because of that, the doctors decided to "fix" the problem, because the guidelines said that the abnormality should be corrected. They gave her large amounts of fluid to lower the abnormally high level of this blood component (creatinine). But the patient's heart could not cope with the additional fluid, and fluid built up in her lungs. As a result, she died—because the doctors were trying to make everything perfect.

Taking a headache pill to relieve a headache and be able to go on with your work is an easy decision. Having surgery for an obstructed bowel needs only a small amount of deliberation. The benefits of treatment are large; the harms are small, or relatively so. The returns are good. The situation gets more difficult as problems become complex, require more effort to correct and have a higher chance of harm. Heart surgery is a good example, as would be chemotherapy for certain cancers. There are specifics and details to consider. In otherwise healthy people, the chances of a favorable outcome are good, but not in someone with multiple medical problems that cannot be fixed.

The odds of a good outcome change quickly and steeply as other health-related concerns come into play. Problems with other systems of the body and advanced age of the patient are two major factors that affect what the outcome could be. It is important to note that the problems don't just add up but actually have a multiplier effect. The complexity, risks and benefits of the proposed treatments obviously need to be weighed. However, if the patient is older and has two or more organs not functioning properly, even relatively minor procedures and treatments can cause problems. The risk/benefit ratio becomes unfavorable, and thereby the law of diminishing returns takes effect. You get less and less benefit, and there is greater and greater risk of serious problems. It is difficult to give exact numbers, exact ratios for how much benefit and risk there is for a patient at the time the problem comes up. But there is a simple point: if you have multiple medical problems, think hard about what benefit a proposed treatment will provide and at what risk.

Your doctor can help, but remember that doctors, in general, tend to do more rather than less. Their training and other factors incline them in that direction. As a patient or a patient's advocate, it is your responsibility to understand the whole situation, the good and the bad. Saying "no" is an acceptable response if the odds are poor. It is your legal right and moral imperative. Think of the whole picture, and accept only those interventions that are likely to benefit you.

Guidelines are helpful, but they must be put into the context of the patient's condition. Otherwise, they may cause harm from over-treatment.

There is another problem with guidelines that has been addressed in a book from Dartmouth Medical School, *Overdiagnosed*. This book analyzes the way guidelines for high blood pressure and diabetes were written and points out the conflict of interest for some of those who wrote the guidelines.[16] Among the experts who drafted the guidelines were physicians who were receiving funds from companies that manufacture drugs for the treatment of diabetes and high blood pressure. Similar helpful guidelines have been written for many diseases in different stages of the spectrum. However, most of them talk about giving more treatments and do not take into account the patient's other health problems or age. Comfort care is mentioned in these guidelines as a last resort when all other options have failed. This attitude transfers to many doctors.

In 2013, the Society for Critical Care Medicine put out their version of "Choosing Wisely." This does mention that patients who are unlikely to benefit from treatment in the ICU should be given comfort care rather than active treatments; this is a positive step. An article in the *New England Journal of Medicine* discusses how it is possible to be in the ICU and still be given comfort care and die with dignity.[17] It provides guidelines for communication and making joint decisions between patients and doctors. This is a step in the right direction, but it is not being followed by most physicians.

BELIEF IN CERTAIN TREATMENTS

Even the most rational person has personal beliefs and superstitions. Sometimes these are irrational; Einstein had some despite his genius, the great work he did and the great ideas he had. Doctors in general are rational. They understand anatomy, physiology, pathology and the like. They look at data and base their decisions on logic and rational analysis.

Sometimes, however, physicians develop a belief system that may not be based wholly on data and rational analysis. Despite evidence to the contrary, they may have an approach to diagnosis or treatment that is rooted in their own thinking. Some may refuse to give up performing a treatment that has been proven by more recent studies to be ineffective. (Maybe some of their patients recovered after receiving the treatment, but these individuals may have gotten better despite, rather than because of, it.) Some may embrace new treatments based on their own analysis of information that has no factual basis.

As in the case of radical mastectomy, some doctors may continue outdated treatments despite evidence to the contrary. For example, until recently some gynecologists routinely removed their patients' healthy uteruses after meno-pause, reasoning that this organ no longer had a reproductive function and might become diseased. These aberrant actions are watched by the doctors' peers, and, if needed, the doctors are counseled appropriately, but such treat-ments still occur much too often. Radical surgeries for cancers of organs like the lung and pancreas are still being performed by some surgeons. It is not a clear-cut issue, but what is clear is that even if the cancer is "cured," the patient can suffer long-term debilitating effects from the surgery.

As a patient, you owe it to yourself to ask your doctors whether the treat-ment they are suggesting is based on solid data and whether the proposed action is in your best interest. I have a friend Dave who has a rare type of inherited disease in which the patient gets multiple, usually slow-growing tumors in the pancreas and the liver. Steve Jobs, the late founder of Apple, had this.[18] When Dave first saw a doctor, he was told that the gold standard for his condition was radical surgery and that he should have it. It may be the "gold standard," but it is not curative, and there are many ongoing problems after the surgery. The gold standard is based on attempts to remove the organs where the tumors occur most commonly—not on consideration of the patient's qual-ity of life after the surgery. Dave refused the radical surgery and has chosen instead to have these tumors removed when they cause him problems. The process is not easy, but he feels he has a better quality of life than he would have had with the recommended "gold standard."

I have a colleague who believes that more treatment is better than less. Even though studies have shown that three treatments are just as good as four or more and that the risks are increased if more treatments are given, he insists on recommending more treatments. His recommendations have, on some occasions, led to severe complications in patients without giving them any benefit. Such beliefs are one of the reasons doctors over-treat.

Having a personal belief is fine, but a doctor's beliefs should not cause harm to patients.

9

Why Doctors Over-Treat

Pressure from Society and the Medical Establishment

Pressure from society in general and from the medical system specifically leads many providers to over-treat. These pressures are subtle, but physicians feel them in many ways when they interact with patients. Some of the more common pressures are as follows:

a. Competitiveness and ambition
b. Specialization
c. Use of the ICU and CPR
d. Fear of lawsuits
e. Personal or employer financial incentives (the Medical Industrial Complex)
f. Research

COMPETITIVENESS AND AMBITION

Doctors are by nature competitive. They competed against their peers to get the best grades in high school and college. Only those with drive and ambition got into medical school. In medical school, they were pitted against people who were, like them, competitive and ambitious. To get into training programs was again hard, because now the young doctors were competing with people from all over the country. It goes on in this manner in all stages of medical studies, in training and in jobs after the training. Doctors remain competitive and ambitious throughout their lives and careers. They show their competitiveness in different ways depending on where they work and what they do.

Jobs and positions of responsibility are structured in the form of a pyramid. The higher you go, the fewer the positions and the greater the competition for them. Of course, there are privileges and benefits at the top—that is why some people strive for those positions. Ambition clouds their judgment and may even lead some doctors to act in ways that are unethical. They have a drive; they feel they must do better than everyone else. But it is *they* who decide what is "better." Despite their "high" positions, they may feel inadequate and need to prove themselves over and over again. Many of them copy ideas or advance half-baked ideas as their own. They also do not want to be less than anyone else. If "A" is doing this, my institution must do it, too. Because they have power, these "top docs" persuade those under them to undertake procedures and treatments that have prestige value but no benefit for the patient.

Competitiveness has many positive aspects, but undertaking medical treatments that are not of proven value, just for the sake of being competitive, is not one of them, and such actions have a high chance of hurting the patient. This is a common phenomenon. Unfortunately, financial gain for the institution and the individual physician also drives them to do more. Medical facilities invest in self-promotion, just like other companies do. The competitiveness of the institution also affects the doctors working there. The two feed on each other, creating an environment that leads to over-treatment.

Doctors compare themselves to other doctors. If they find that another doctor is performing a particular procedure or undertaking a new treatment, they often feel compelled to "keep up." Many times they try that procedure without a complete understanding of the circumstances, the full background or the good and the bad that may result. They may feel that they would be considered behind the times if they didn't offer the new treatment. This is another cause of unnecessary treatments.

When bone marrow transplantation was advocated by the "experts" at some major universities as a treatment for breast cancer, every hospital that was capable of doing the procedure jumped on the bandwagon. They had a double incentive to be copy-cat transplant centers. First, there had been a lawsuit in California that forced insurance companies to reimburse hospitals fully for the cost of the transplantation. The hospitals could charge exorbitant fees, and they pushed many patients into bone marrow transplants for certain types of breast cancer. There was a profit to be made. On top of that, the hospital and the oncologist could boast that they were offering the state-of-the-art treatments.

It so happened that due to the well-publicized unethical behavior of one doctor in South Africa, it became clear that bone marrow transplantation was not a useful procedure except in very few diseases—none of them forms of breast cancer.[1] The South African study was not the only one that demonstrated lack of efficacy; many others did. But investigation of the shoddy ethics of those physicians brought the problem to public attention, and insurance companies stopped paying for bone marrow transplantation for breast cancer. The procedure was discontinued, and many oncologists and hospitals lost money and prestige.

It is not just individual doctors, but hospitals and medical centers that are competitive. They do not want to be left behind. If "A" has a new piece of equipment, "B" will get it too. They will train someone to use that equipment, which is supposed to be better. Now that they have paid for the equipment and spent money training the personnel, they have to recover their costs. They obtained the equipment to be competitive, not necessarily to help their patients. They need to advertise their newest, latest advance. When they get patients on whom the equipment is used, they bill the patients for the services and for part of the cost of the equipment. This is how they recoup their investment in the technology, and that is the reality of the fee-for-service medical system. The degree of benefit that the patients get from the new equipment and procedure is not necessarily the main reason to obtain and use the equipment. A hospital in my area had a billboard saying: *We don't treat cancer. We cure it.* A misleading claim.

Hospitals and medical centers function on a business model. The publicity put out by those institutions emphasizes their high-tech capabilities. Like ads produced by other commercial entities, the ads for hospitals and medical institutions use selective stories to give the impression that they can solve problems that no one else could—misleading and unfortunate hype. There is a national network of five hospitals in the United States that advertises regularly on TV and in magazines. They emphasize how one in two men and one in three women will be diagnosed with cancer during their lifetimes and that one in eight cancer patients are misdiagnosed. While these statements are accurate in themselves, they do not mention that these numbers include many cancers that have no significant effect on the patient's life. They promise "precision cancer treatments" for your cancer. The reality is that only a small number of cancers need such "precision" evaluation and treatment. Yes, gene-based cancer therapy can be of value for a small number of patients, but these are few, and the benefits are marginal. However, these advertisements convince patients to come to these centers and thus increase their business. Of course, they put in small print the disclaimer "No case is typical. You should not expect to experience these results."

Competitiveness has the advantage of keeping a physician, a clinic, a hospital or a medical center abreast of the latest advances. The patient, however, may have difficulty deciding if the competitive behavior is for medical reasons or for business reasons. As a patient, you should ask questions and satisfy yourself as to what is in your own best interest.

A nurse from the world-famous Johns Hopkins Medical Center once pointed out that she had never seen a hospital that advertises compassion and comfort as their strength. They are focused on "advances," and that mind-set is pervasive. Doctors are encouraged to try treatments that may not be in the patient's best interest; the institution functions this way, and so do the doctors working there.

SPECIALIZATION

Medical science has made many advances. We understand the normal working of the body much more clearly than we did even just a few years ago. We also have more tools to treat the problems that do occur. One of the reasons for this newer and better understanding is the specialization that has occurred in the physicians' training. The ability to understand in depth one area of the body or one type of disease has benefits. By the nature of their training, specialists understand and know more about a particular organ or illness. A cardiologist will comprehend more aspects of heart function than a general physician; similarly a specialist in infectious disease will understand infections more clearly than other doctors, and an oncologist will know more about cancer than her colleagues in other fields. Specialists are very important, even essential, for the delivery of good medical care.

These days, there are many physicians and other health-care providers who are specialists. After their general training, they receive further training in a specialty and become nephrologists (kidney doctors), psychiatrists (behavioral health doctors), orthopedists (bone and joint surgeons) and so on.

Their perspective is dominated by their training and experience in their area of expertise—at which they are very good. Neurologists, neurosurgeons, cancer surgeons, psychiatrists and many other specialists are excellent at what they do. I would take advantage of their special knowledge and skills if I were in need of them. However, specialized doctors live and breathe their specialties. Their perspective with regard to the patient as a whole may be limited. It brings to mind the common saying "To a hammer, everything is a nail." The input of the specialist can be helpful in difficult situations; however, it should be only one part of a total picture of what ails the patient. Too often, it is not.

The downside to specialization is its focus on one aspect of the patient's condition at the cost of ignoring the patient's other problems. It is not uncommon for each specialist to think of the patient as "a kidney" or "a heart." What is lost is what happens if heart and kidney are both damaged. The two organs, and others in the body, are interconnected. Someone needs to keep an eye on the whole person. This is when the generalist is more helpful.

A common scenario is that of a specialist who assesses the patient for a specific problem. For example, a kidney specialist is consulted because a blood test suggests the kidneys are not functioning normally. The nephrologist knows how to fix that problem. But the patient may also have a damaged heart, mental deterioration or stroke, and the correction of the kidney abnormality revealed by the blood report is not going to help him. The patient, not the tests, should be the center point of decision-making. The recommendations from the medical team should be those that improve the patient's overall welfare. Specialists often forget this.

The key decisions regarding tests, and especially treatments with a major impact, should be made by the patient and a physician who has an understanding of the whole patient. The specialists should work with the generalist (the patient's primary care physician) but often do not. One specialist, after her assessment, may talk to the patient and family and explain what is wrong with the organ she is expert in. The specialist suggests ways of fixing that problem. Another problem is looked at by another specialist, who discusses what can be done for that one. Each specialist discusses the problem and solutions from his or her point of view. The family gets hope that this or that can be controlled or fixed.

However, when the physicians who take care of the patient explain the *total* picture, the family may be confused. The generalist physician looks at the holistic picture and the inter-relationship between the different body systems and tries to present the realistic scenario. Often because of the discussions with the specialists, the patient and family are unable to accept the reality of the patient's full state of health. Our society tends to give a higher ranking to specialists, and patients' hopes can be heightened because of what the specialists told them. The explanation of the overall medical reality is hard for them to accept. Specialists are essential for advances in medicine in general and for the care of individual patients. Yet the fragmented analyses and lack of communication with the generalist about the problems can cause difficulties.

Why are specialists given more importance in our society? This is an interesting question and may be looked upon as a spiral where more begets more. Let me start with a comment I remember from my high school days (*many* years ago): "A specialist is one who knows more and more about less and less—until he knows everything about nothing." Specialists train for three to five more years after medical school than those who do not specialize. They get new knowledge and skills, which they apply to the treatment of patients and to research. These doctors feel they deserve extra compensation for their specialized knowledge and for the extra years they spent in training. Society and the system seem to agree. Specialists are paid more than non-specialists. Because of the focus of their work, they can do a very good job. Take, for example, surgeons who only do knee replacements or cataract surgery. They are trained, they do one thing, and they do it well, benefiting from experience as they do the same procedure over and over. They also make good money—very good money. They have no concerns other than knees or cataracts.

Then there are specialists who learn more and more about, say, heart disease. They sub-specialize and learn even more about one type of heart disease. The point is they work with patients with a particular disease. They do not, by nature of their work and training, look at the whole patient or the patient's other medical problems. They only consider the problems related to their area of expertise. In addition to being well-compensated, they often are interviewed by the media and become local celebrities. When they express an opinion, it carries a lot of weight. The generalist, who is one of many in the system, is not considered that important—even though it is the generalist who keeps everything together and who probably knows the patient longest and best.

Specialists also get a lot of additional recognition because many philanthropists and advocacy groups prefer to fund specific, focused types of research.

With their training and focus on one area, specialists can sway many patients, families and even other doctors to undertake treatments that may control the disease but not help the patient. It has been said that specialists get more bucks for their bang while generalists get more bang for their bucks.

Partly as a result of their focus, doctors, especially specialists, keep trying to do more. They want to do their best, and they are likely to do more rather than less. Given that (understandable) bias, patients and their families should recognize that if a physician says that nothing more can be done, it really does mean that nothing more can be done to control the disease process that is causing the patient to be sick. The goal at this point needs to change to the patient's comfort.

Problems arise because of specialization in the hospital, where the patient may be seen by multiple specialists, in addition to his generalist. Multiple specialists make sure that all that can or needs to be done to evaluate and treat appropriately is being done. However, an unfortunate scenario has been described to me by medical students when I meet with them to discuss problems they have noted during their hospital rotations. Those sessions allow the students to describe, anonymously, what they saw and heard that troubled them. We have a large number of patients in our hospital who have badly damaged livers due to excessive alcohol intake. Many of these patients continue their drinking despite being informed of the heightened risks of alcohol in the presence of liver damage. These patients can be very sick, and often their cognitive function is impaired because their faulty livers are allowing poisons to affect their brains.

What the students have described is that the primary team taking care of the patient, who sees the patient as a whole, is concerned that the patient's overall condition is getting worse according to his blood counts, clinical picture and mental capacity. Members of the primary care team try to explain to the patient and family the grave situation they are in. But the liver specialists come to see the patient and look only at the liver tests. It may happen that on a given day, the numbers may have improved compared to the previous day. The hepatologist (liver specialist) looks at that one test and gives the family (the patient may be too confused to understand) hope by saying that "things look better." But the hope the family develops is false hope. The reality is that overall even the liver tests are not showing that the patient is improving. This focused, partial assessment hurts the patient because it will be harder for him to accept that he is getting worse and will most likely die soon. The hepatologist was being optimistic and had a narrow perspective, but his opinion carried more weight because he was a specialist. The generalist was being a realist and had a broader understanding of the patient as a whole human being. Consultation with a specialist may be in order, but the total picture should not be forgotten by the patient and family or by the doctors.

In her book *Knocking on Heaven's Door*, Katy Butler describes the problems she and her mother faced when dealing with her father's illness.[2] He was in his eighties, had suffered a large stroke and also had a heart condition. Their primary physician, who made his recommendations after assessing the whole patient, said that heart surgery was not in her father's best interest. The heart specialist only looked at the problems in the heart and suggested surgery. The family (the patient was cognitively impaired and could not make decisions) agreed with the internist and refused the surgery, a decision they were happy with. Butler also describes, in some detail, the problems that her mother was facing because she, also in her eighties, was the main caregiver for her husband.

We would do well to remember the old adage about physicians: "He who knows only one branch of his arts is like a bird with one wing."

USE OF THE ICU AND CPR

An ICU is an important part of medical treatment of severely ill patients. The ICU is staffed by highly trained doctors and other health professionals who monitor and treat patients who might not survive without their expertise and interventions. The team works around the clock, striving to bring their patients through acute crises. Sometimes patients die despite these efforts, but ICU doctors (now called intensivists) focus on saving lives from immediate threats, not on giving patients a comfortable death.

There are ICUs for babies, children and adults. There are ICUs for patients who undergo difficult surgery, those who have suffered severe injury or burns, and those who have had injury to the brain or a severe heart attack. Each of these specialized facilities provides patients with support and help that are often not possible outside the ICU. There is, however, a simple premise to justify treating a patient in the ICU. The patient's problem has to be a process that is reversible and temporary in nature—for example, the patient has a severe pneumonia preventing her lungs from supplying enough oxygen

to her body, or the patient has lost a large amount of blood or fluids and cannot nourish his body or his brain. In such situations, the ICU can save many
lives, but treatments in the ICU cannot repair damaged organs or organs that
have been taken over by cancer cells. Some patients are simply too sick for
the ICU.

Age per se is not a deciding factor in medical decision-making. But it is well
known that older patients heal more slowly and recover with more difficulty
after surgery or infections. Recovery and survival of elderly patients after ICU
treatments is also limited. A study of older patients who were treated in the
ICU found that one-third of very elderly ICU patients died in hospital, many
after prolonged ICU stay while continuing to receive aggressive life-sustaining
interventions. These findings raise questions about the use of critical care at
the end of life for the very elderly.[3]

Patients in the ICU are very ill, and this leads to a lot of tension among
patients, families and medical providers. Careful, sensitive discussion among
all parties is essential. Although communication and open and frank conversation are always helpful, they are crucial when the patient is very sick and a
decision about treatment in the ICU needs to be made. Sometimes patients
with long-standing irreversible illnesses are put in the ICU, seemingly with the
expectation that they will be better off there. This practice does not help the
patient. It only causes distress to the patient, to the family and to those who
work in the ICU. A colleague of mine pointed out a simple fact: The ICU is a
bridge to good health. If the patient is very sick with multiple medical problems, the ICU becomes a bridge from nowhere to nowhere. For a patient in
the final stages of a serious illness, the ICU can make the line between life and
death fuzzy. Treatment there just prolongs the process of dying.

End-of-life discussion, if clear and honest, reduces the number of patients
that are transferred to the ICU. One study showed that a third of the patients
with advanced cancer who were in the ICU did not know why they were there
and what the goal of treatment was.[4]

Patients with no chance of recovery should not be in the ICU. They are
taking up a precious bed, causing stress for the medical providers and wasting
resources. (Because of the high technology and highly trained staff involved,
doctors and nurses sometimes call the ICU the "Expensive Care Unit.")
Resources that could be used on a patient who *can* benefit from being in the
ICU are expended on those who cannot. Sometimes patients who *can* benefit

from ICU treatments have to be taken hundreds of miles away because all ICU beds in their area are occupied, many of them by patients who will not recover and should be receiving comfort care.

The dramatic recovery of some patients who were appropriately in the ICU has created a false impression that every patient should have the option of treatment in the ICU—that this is the place where any seriously ill patient will receive the *best* care. Many people believe that if they are not treated in the ICU, they are not getting all the benefits that modern medicine has to offer. This is not the case. Yes, at times, in unclear situations, patients may be given a trial of treatment in the ICU, but if it does not result in improvement, the best course of action is to stop the intensive treatment and to provide comfort to the patient. Even though it is called the intensive "care" unit, in reality, it is really an intensive *treatment* unit. Lights are always on, monitors beep, and staff hurry to and from bedsides, checking on patients and conducting tests at all hours. Comfort care is best delivered outside that bustling setting. The difference between "care" and "treatment" is important to remember, but it often is forgotten.

Let us look more specifically and compare some of the treatments that may be used in the time before death and how they contrast with a plan to use measures to make you comfortable. In the ICU, you will need to be on monitors that will record your heart rate, your blood pressure and how much oxygen your body is getting. Monitors are electric devices that are either connected to your body by an electric pad or put into your artery or vein. Most monitors have a light and beeper that flash or beep according to the various parameters they are measuring, such as with your heart beat or when whatever the monitor is measuring goes above or below a set level. This informs the nurses and doctors, and they respond as needed. The monitors are essential for the medical personnel to know the condition of your body, but the beeping and flashing are not conducive to your rest and comfort. Also, of course, if there is a change in the readings, the nurses and doctors have to come in and take corrective action.

If the treatment in the ICU has a reasonable chance of making you better, this discomfort is justified and appropriate. If it is just to placate a false hope, it is only making your precious last days of life difficult. A friend of mine had a very severe attack of asthma. She was placed in the ICU to monitor her condition because any further worsening would have required putting a tube down her throat to provide adequate amounts of oxygen to her body. She did not need the tube and recovered sufficiently with the help of medications that were given to her that she could be moved within 24 hours to the regular medical floor of the hospital and was discharged from the hospital the following day. The ICU had helped bring her through the acute crisis, which is what it was meant to do.

My friend is smart and observant and a writer. She said she had discomfort from the asthma but also described the experience of being in the ICU. What struck her most was how intrusive and noisy it was and how little peace and comfort she had. Although she could doze off, she was never able to sleep. She confirmed that it was an intensive *treatment* unit and not an intensive *care* unit. As she was wheeled out to her regular room, she noticed that most, perhaps all, of the other ICU patients she passed appeared to be near death.

I participated in a discussion regarding a 52-year-old man. The ICU doctors were discussing with the family the futility of continuing treatment of this patient there. His lungs were damaged, and two weeks of ICU treatments had produced no improvement in their condition. In addition, he had lung cancer that had spread to his brain. The brain had been radiated in an attempt to shrink the cancer, but the radiation had not resulted in any improvement. The lung cancer itself was not treatable.

In light of these multiple problems for which there were no effective treatments, the doctors wanted to move the man out of the ICU and allow him to die in peace. There was no possible way to control any of his major disease processes. However, the family would not accept the doctors' advice and recommendations—somewhat understandably because of the patient's relatively young age. Although the doctors were totally justified in discontinuing treatments that were not going to make the patient better, they were reluctant to override the family's wishes; so they continued treatment in the ICU. What were the reasons why the doctors were unable to stop the painful, futile treatments? After all, these treatments also caused moral distress to those involved in treating, rather than caring for, the patient. Why did they not override the family's irrational demand?

The prevailing belief is that the hospital's administration would not have supported overriding the family's wishes and facing the negative publicity that could have ensued if the family complained to the media. Through subtle pressure, a hospital's administration controls the actions of the doctors who work there, especially if what a doctor recommends falls outside the realm of active treatments. I know of a university medical center that did not allow a member of the faculty to hold a seminar on "choices at the end of life." Their stated reason was that the topic was "controversial." The implication was that the discussion would include less treatment and more emphasis on comfort care. Fear of lawsuits was also cited as a reason. As described in the next section, this is not a justified fear. If the medical facts are clear and well-documented, the chances of a lawsuit are close to zero, but the fear persists. If the situation is sympathetically and honestly explained, the family is likely to agree to discontinuing intensive treatments. The issue of overriding the patient's wishes is discussed in chapter 11: "When Doctors Say 'No.'"

In 2015, the *American Journal of Respiratory and Critical Care Medicine* published a policy statement from multiple associations and societies whose members are involved with treatments of patients who are in the ICU. They recommend communication and ethics consultations to help reduce conflict. But they also state: If the treatment is "truly futile—meaning that it simply cannot accomplish its physiological aims—clinicians should refuse to administer the treatment."[5]

Related to treatment in the ICU is the issue of CPR (heart-lung resuscitation). CPR refers to reviving the function of a heart that has stopped beating. The process also forces oxygen into the lungs, so that they can deliver it to the heart, brain and other vital organs. Thus, CPR is a treatment given *after* the heart has stopped—the person is dead. There are many reasons for the heart to stop beating. Sometimes it stops because of a drug overdose, a major heart attack or a severe electrical shock. Most commonly, however, the heart stops after the body has given out and life cannot be sustained. It is the last event in the process of dying.

This medical use of CPR is the one that is relevant here—not the CPR that a lifeguard may give at the water's edge to a drowning victim he has rescued or that a mother trained in first aid might utilize to save the life of her child who has choked on a peppermint. In rare cases such as these, the heart stops beating even though the rest of the body is still functioning and reasonably healthy. If the heart of a fairly healthy person stops, there is some chance that CPR will restore heart function and the patient may survive. However, if the heart stops because the rest of the body has given out, the chances of restoring a heartbeat are very small, and even if it is restored, it lasts for a short time.

Since the body is not functioning, restoring the heartbeat for a short time is of no benefit to the patient.

Under current practice, all patients in the hospital are supposed to undergo CPR if their hearts stop beating. This practice is considered to be the default action since the 1950s. It is required unless a specific decision is made in advance *not* to undertake CPR. Ideally, the decision to forego CPR is made after discussion and agreement between the patient (and/or family) and the doctor responsible for the patient's treatment and care. As described above, if the patient has damaged vital organs, CPR is not likely to be successful and, even if successful, provides no benefit. Therefore, it should not be undertaken. This discussion is an essential part of planning and decision-making.

During the hospital or clinic registration process, it is customary to record the "code status" of the patient, whereby patients state their choice of what they want done if their hearts were to stop beating. "Full code" means that they would like the doctors to try to revive the heartbeat. If they do not want the doctors to revive the heartbeat, they can say "Do Not Resuscitate" (DNR). This is good. Unfortunately, often this information is collected by a clerk who may not fully understand the meaning of the terms.

This information is also confirmed by a nurse or doctor in the hospital. Frequently, however, full details of the implication of the decision are not explained to the patient.

Sometimes the doctors feel that a full code is not in the patient's best interest because of the patient's poor medical condition and because it would not work. Rather than explaining the reality of the situation to the patient, I have regularly seen doctors trying to frighten the patient into accepting DNR. The information they provide is in itself accurate. Trying to revive the heartbeat is a painful process.

What is not explained to the patient is that because she has multiple, chronic and irreversible conditions, the attempts to revive the heart will not work and certainly will not fix the underlying problems. I feel it is the doctor's responsibility to give all the information to the patient. In fact, since I work with advanced cancer patients, I make it a point to explain the futility and lack of benefit of attempts to revive the heartbeat in situations like theirs. The same applies for other coexisting multiple diseases. I explain the reality and then make a *recommendation* to the patient to give permission for a DNR order.

When I communicate this clearly and sympathetically, patients accept the reality. Of course, this has to be combined with the explanation that all other needed treatments will be continued and the patient and loved ones will not be abandoned.

In case your heart stops beating and you have not specifically rejected CPR, the procedures the doctors, nurses or emergency medical technicians (EMTs) (if you are at home and someone calls "911") have to undertake to restore the heartbeat are extremely painful; some call them brutal. (This process is far more extreme than the manual CPR that lay people learn in first aid class and use, for example, to revive near-drowning victims.) The heart needs to be brought back to normal rhythmic beating. This requires either electric shocks to the heart or a large amount of mechanical pressure on the heart, which necessitates compressing the chest wall and ribs. It is quite common for some ribs to be broken in the process. At the same time, in order to provide adequate amounts of oxygen to the body, a tube has to be inserted down the patient's windpipe, a painful procedure in itself. Then oxygen is pushed into the lungs under pressure. If this is likely to restore the body to a functioning status for a reasonable amount of time, it may be worthwhile to suffer through that pain. But if the chance is minimal that the patient will survive and be reasonably functional, is it worth it?

Treatment in the ICU and with CPR most often deprives the patient of a chance to be comfortable, with no benefit despite the pain of the procedures.

Accepting and understanding the realities of what CPR means will help reduce your distress as you decide whether to reject it in advance. The success of CPR is grossly misrepresented to the public, especially by the media. In a survey of TV shows, they depicted that CPR was successful in 75 percent of cases and that 65 percent of patients went home after successful CPR.[6] The misrepresentation of the success of CPR was confirmed by another study looking at the popular shows *Grey's Anatomy* and *House*. Jaclyn Portanova and her colleagues found that 69.6 percent of 46 CPR attempts depicted were successful and 71.9 percent of those fictional patients survived to be discharged from the hospital.[7] The study also noted that advance directive discussions occurred for only two patients and preferences for code status, intubation and feeding occurred in fewer than 10 percent of the situations. TV shows and films continue to give an unrealistic picture, sending the wrong message and misleading the public.

The reality is that fewer than 10 percent of patients survive for more than a month after successful CPR. Further, only about 3 percent can lead a normal life.[8] The odds are even worse if the patient had poor health prior to the CPR. Do not be swayed by the false picture given by medical melodramas. Think, discuss with your doctor and put a DNR order in your chart. DNR does not mean "Do Not Care." If anything, such an order increases the "care" that you will get. Another way to look at this situation is to think of it as Allowing Natural Death (AND).

FEAR OF LAWSUITS

The legal system and the medical system both have a lot to offer to individuals and the community as a whole. They work together to create regulations and laws that are helpful to everyone. Lawyers protect the users of the health-care system and make sure that the public and patients are receiving what is due to them. They ensure that Medicare and Medicaid benefits are available to those who qualify. They watch over insurance companies, drug manufacturers and those who make medical devices. They also work to reduce fraud in whatever form it occurs. In hospitals and in different types of medical centers, lawyers and doctors work together to ensure that all patients receive legal protection—as in the case of immigrants or underprivileged people. They make sure there are appropriate policies in place for the protection of those in need and that these are enforced. They also help protect the personnel from the inappropriate behavior of patients. The expertise of these professionals, when they work together, is of benefit to all.

At times, disagreements arise between doctors and patients about what treatments should or should not have been given. At other times, mistakes are made or the patient feels that mistakes were made. In most cases, discussions, explanations and communication, when carried out openly and honestly, resolve the problem. The doctors acknowledge the mistake or explain why the patient thought there was a mistake when there was none. Explanation is given as to why a treatment was or was not undertaken. Such open conversation usually brings about better understanding of the situation.

Unfortunately, for a variety of reasons, sometimes the disagreement persists and can go on to become a "dispute." In order to protect herself and to seek redemption or compensation, the patient may file a lawsuit against the providers. An adversarial relationship develops. Even in these cases, the two sides work together and try to resolve the differences and develop an understanding with each other. This process is facilitated in some cases by a neutral panel of doctors and lawyers who work together to look into the details of the dispute and evaluate the circumstances of the case. If there is a reasonable possibility that there was a medical error, they advise whether it might have resulted in any actual harm. Despite these efforts, sometimes the dispute is not resolved. Then the judicial system gets involved, and juries decide the merits of the case. The process of a legal dispute, from the filing of a lawsuit to its resolution, is stressful to the doctor. Understandably, doctors want to prevent this as much as they can.

To avoid the unpleasantness and cost of lawsuits, an approach commonly used by doctors is to practice what is called "defensive medicine." They conduct tests and treatments that they know are not really needed. A survey of doctors in different parts of the country and of doctors practicing different specialties has found that around 70 to 80 percent had practiced defensive medicine.[9] They do the tests just to protect themselves in the event of a dispute. For example, a patient has a minor head trauma. After examining the individual, the doctor concludes that there is no reasonable chance of damage to the brain and the patient will be fine. Despite the medical evaluation, which shows that there is no need for a CT scan of the head, the doctor orders the test anyway, "just in case." Just in case—not because of suspicion of brain injury, but just in case the patient may file a lawsuit. There are many examples of these tests and procedures being done "just in case."

The reasons why doctors are so concerned about lawsuits are complex. Some of their information is based on incidents they have heard about. They have heard that one doctor was sued by a patient's family and the legal process had a major impact on the doctor's life, professional reputation and emotional health, even though it was ruled that he had done no wrong. Stories of that nature make all physicians inclined to do too much to minimize the chances of being sued.

However, research on medical malpractice lawsuits has shown that most result from actual negligence. "Frivolous" lawsuits are the exception. Plaintiff's lawyers, the legal specialists who represent the allegedly injured party, accept cases only after deciding there is a good chance of showing that there was negligence that resulted in harm. This is because plaintiff's lawyers generally work on contingency; their only payment is a percentage of what their clients receive. They make no money if the case has no merit; they don't even make back their out-of-pocket expenses, which can range from Xeroxing documents to paying fees to experts. If as a patient you feel you have been harmed because of negligence, discuss your complaint with your doctor. If you are not satisfied, you have the right to sue.

One of the reasons for lawsuits is that through our hype and overemphasis on advances in medical achievements, we have raised the expectations of the public. This false hope and subsequent disappointment make some people feel that if the outcome is not what they hoped and expected, the right treatment was not given, and they sue the doctors. For example, if a baby is born with birth defects, rather than accepting that not all newborns are perfect, the parents may conclude that the obstetrician who conducted the delivery did something wrong. Assuming that they can find a lawyer to take the case, they may file a lawsuit.

In addition, certain vested interests overplay the impact of medical malpractice suits by publicizing the high-profile, though rare, cases. Malpractice insurance companies try to take advantage of the fear generated by such lawsuits, raising premiums and fees. The main benefit of such publicity often goes to the insurance companies. Defensive medicine causes a significant waste of money and other resources. Many policy-makers and organizations are trying to find ways to reduce this waste, but it is a complicated and difficult issue.[10]

Even though the likelihood of actually being sued is quite low, providers still operate in the shadow and fear of lawsuits.[11] It is not the fear of making a wrong diagnosis, but the fear of a lawsuit that leads to the unnecessary tests and treatments—to doctors doing too much. It is not possible to say how often and to what degree this phenomenon occurs, but it unfortunately seems to be all too frequent. Defensive medicine does not help patients, doctors, the medical system or society. But it occurs. From the patients' viewpoint, they could ask the doctors if the test is really needed, but this does not happen too often. Proper and complete evaluation including tests that are appropriate is a part of good medical care. Defensive medicine is not.

Attempts have been made to reduce medical malpractice lawsuits as well as to reduce defensive medicine. An article by Daniel Waxman of the University of California, Los Angeles, and several colleagues in the *New England Journal of Medicine* reported that despite malpractice reform (including limits on how much doctors would pay if they lost a case), the practice of defensive medicine did not decrease.[12] Unneeded tests and treatments continued. The fear of lawsuits is deeply ingrained, and young doctors absorb it from their senior colleagues.

Doctors and lawyers agree that communication and documentation are more effective in reducing the chances of a lawsuit than defensive medicine. If the doctor explains to the patient why she is *not* doing a CT scan and documents her reasons, the chances of a lawsuit are very small. If doctors explain to patients, in clear language, what the disease is, what treatments are available and how likely they are to help, the patient will usually be satisfied. Such clear conversation is the best way to reduce the chances of a malpractice lawsuit. If there is a complication and the doctors openly explain the full story, the chances of the patient suing the doctor decrease markedly. Patients understand that anyone can make a mistake, that not all diseases can be cured and that not all problems can be fixed. If the doctor shows due respect for the patient and is courteous and honest, the chance of a lawsuit will be negligible.

Further, if the doctor documents the facts, his reasoning and the discussion with the patient, even if there is a lawsuit, it is likely to go in the doctor's favor. Promptly writing down a summary of the discussion and what tests or treatments were given (or not given) and why helps in case there is a lawsuit. The doctor should not give in to the temptation to do too much just because the patient wants it; medical judgment must be given due credibility.

PERSONAL OR EMPLOYER FINANCIAL INCENTIVES (THE MEDICAL INDUSTRIAL COMPLEX)

Medical doctors do not work in isolation. Most are associated with some kind of institution or group. Drugs and devices are a significant part of their work. With that, they have relationships with drug companies and manufacturers of medical devices. We need to understand doctors' interactions with medical institutions and manufacturers to understand the actions that lead them to do too much for financial gain or fame. We will look closely at these components separately and inter-relatedly. In 1980 Arnold Relman, former editor of the *New England Journal of Medicine*, coined the term "Medical Industrial Complex."[13] He was drawing an analogy from the term "Military Industrial Complex" used by President Dwight Eisenhower in his farewell address to the country at the end of his term, explaining how some industries had distorted and taken over the nation's defense.

There are three components of the Medical Industrial Complex.

1. Doctors
2. Medical institutions
3. Drug companies and manufacturers of medical devices

Doctors

It is possible for doctors to earn extra money in many different ways. They could conduct unnecessary tests (especially if they have a financial interest in the laboratory or imaging facility). To decide what constitutes an unnecessary test is very difficult. The medical standards for when or how frequently a test should be done are not defined, so it is most often the doctor's call. But it has been noted that if doctors have a financial interest in a laboratory, they tend to do more tests and more frequently. A study published in the *Annals of Internal Medicine* found that $500 million was spent because of overuse of tests.[14] Extra money can also be made by giving more treatments in their offices or clinics or in hospitals owned wholly or partly by the doctors. Again, it is difficult to define what is "extra," but some doctors have been questioned because they were very much out of line with their peers.

In some cases, doctors pay for the drugs they buy; the drug is then either administered by the doctor or by a nurse who works with the doctor, and there is a markup.[15] The system is complicated, but, as a generalization, it can be said that the doctors receive a percentage of the cost of a drug. In actual dollar amounts, the more expensive the drug, the more they get paid. Doctors often prescribe more expensive drugs when cheaper drugs would be just as efficacious. They may even prescribe drugs that are not really needed.

In April 2014, Medicare released data on doctors' billing practices that described many instances of overbilling.[16] What was most striking were payments to ophthalmologists. One doctor received $11.8 million for the use of an expensive drug injected into the eye. If an equally effective but cheaper drug had been used, the payment would have been $500,000—more than twentyfold less. Medicare and the Affordable Care Act are attempting to fix such problems.

As described earlier, chronic renal (kidney) dialysis can keep many patients functioning if their kidneys have failed. Unfortunately, many patients who are not functional because of other medical problems are dialyzed regularly even though the dialysis does not help them feel any better. There is a strong reason to believe that some receive dialysis because the doctors are paid for performing the procedure. Since the 1970s dialysis has been fully covered by Medicare,[17] which is why for-profit dialysis clinics show up in shopping centers even in small towns.

In his recent book, physician Sandeep Jauhar describes how some doctors refer patients to other doctors just to increase their income. They develop a network in which "'A' refers to 'B,' and 'B' in turn refers to 'A.'" This way, both "A" and "B" get extra revenue. Of course, referrals are needed to get the best treatment for the patient. But Jauhar describes a network which just works on the system "You scratch my back and I will scratch your back."[18]

In the field of oncology, chemotherapy as an unacceptable source of income has been brought to light.[19] It is clear that chemotherapy in many cases leads to additional comfort, prolongation of life and even cures, especially for first-line chemotherapy—chemotherapy given when the cancer is first diagnosed. Second-line chemotherapy is usually less effective but may help some patients. Third- and fourth-line chemotherapy is usually not beneficial. Oncologists, however, are fully reimbursed for using third- and fourth-line chemotherapy. In many instances oncologists administer this form of chemotherapy for personal gain. The American Society of Clinical Oncology is now addressing this issue.[20]

Financial gain through over-treatment was demonstrated by a recent study of the method of payment to oncologists in private practice. Traditionally oncologists have made much of their income by marking up the expensive chemotherapy drugs they give in their offices. UnitedHealth Group Inc. (UHG) tried a different method of payment in a study it conducted with five medical groups.[21] It paid the doctors on a per-*patient* basis—a lump sum payment for the treatment of each patient (in contrast to the previous system, where doctors were paid for each treatment). UHG thus removed the incentive to mark up drugs and the temptation to use expensive drugs and ineffective chemotherapy.

In the three years of the study, UHG spent $64.4 million—compared to $98.1 million that would have been spent if the payment had been on a per-*treatment* basis—a 34 percent reduction! This study suggests that financial incentives do play a role in decision-making about chemotherapy and had major implications regarding future payments to doctors and hospitals.

Another study found that in Kansas City, Medicare spent $7,600 for an average enrollee, while in Miami they spent $16,300.[22] The main difference between the two communities was that most doctors in Kansas City were on a salary, while those in Miami were paid for each visit and treatment. The doctors in Kansas City had no financial incentive to over-treat. No one can clearly say if the Miami treatments were justified or not. No one can say for sure if they were wrong. But some doctors do consider personal financial gain when they conduct tests and treatments, and in the process they may do too much. This problem is inherent in our fee-for-service system. Doctors are paid for a patient's visit on the basis of the "billing level." The billing level is determined by what and how much the doctors did. They submit the bill to the insurance company or Medicare and are paid. The payers generally accept the bill the doctor submitted. However, they do periodically carry out audits to verify the billing, and they look at medical records.

The billing levels are labeled 1 through 5, 1 being a short visit for a simple problem and 5 being extensive review of records, detailed history, examination and planning for future tests and treatments. The doctor is expected to document all the components of the encounter. Payment is made based on the documentation which, obviously, is expected to reflect what was *actually* done. One recent report from the Inspector General of Health and Human Services noted that there has been a decrease in billings at levels 1, 2 and 3 while level 4 billings have increased correspondingly.[23] It is possible that doctors are spending more time with their patients and doing a more complete job. Another possible explanation was revealed to me by a medical student. Before entering medical school, the student had worked as a "scribe" at a hospital. When the doctor saw a patient, the scribe entered the categories of the history-taking and examination that the physician conducted. She did this accurately. When the doctor looked at her entries, he was upset. "Why have you not filled all the boxes?" he demanded. The scribe replied that she had filled out what she observed him do. When she saw the final record, she found that all the boxes had been checked. The doctor seemed to have billed for a number of things he had not actually done.

An additional source of personal gain for doctors is by having a direct financial interest in a hospital. Atul Gawande wrote an article reporting that the cost of similar procedures and treatments were three times higher in hospitals that were owned by doctors as compared to public hospitals.[24] Such financial relationships are being examined by different regulatory bodies, and attempts are being made to curb this practice.

The *New Yorker* also ran an article pointing out that by 2005 nearly 10 percent of physicians in the United States had established relationships with the investment industry.[25] This leads to a conflict of interest because physicians make large investments in pharmaceutical companies. They could have inside information that could give them an unfair advantage. The article further describes the insider trading regarding a drug for Alzheimer's disease.

Personal gain that is not connected to direct financial gain is another difficult problem that deserves comment. An obstetrician may order a caesarian section in order to be able to "schedule" a delivery to suit her social schedule, rather than because a vaginal delivery would be medically complicated for mother or baby. Or a surgeon may decide to undertake a procedure because he wants to show that he is capable of successfully performing a new or difficult surgery. It may be unclear whether the procedure is really likely to help the particular patient, so there may be some disagreement even among the surgeon's colleagues about whether this is the right course of action. But, as before, it is appropriate, even necessary, for the patient to have a detailed discussion with the surgeon about the potential benefits and drawbacks of the new surgery.

An unfortunate reality, thankfully rare, is that some doctors undertake tests, procedures or treatments only for personal gain, fully aware that the patient will not benefit and may even be harmed. There are well-known cases of fraud in which the treatment was given just for personal gain. Sometimes, the procedure is not even done, and Medicare or the insurance company is billed. Fraud of this nature is outside the scope of our discussion and is covered by criminal investigators and the judicial system. I have no personal knowledge of such actions, but newspapers describe them on a regular basis. Financial gain, personal glory and a narcissistic mind-set are all reasons why doctors undertake tests and treatments that will not help the patient; these are the most deplorable reasons why doctors do too much.

Medical Institutions

Hospitals, health science centers and specialized clinics all work, and are expected by their boards to work, on a business model. Many of these institutions are classified as "non-profit" organizations. As a result, they are in a special tax category, 501(c), under the rules of the Internal Revenue Service (they pay lesser amounts in taxes), and they are allowed to accept tax-deductible donations from individuals or businesses. They can also hold fundraisers of different kinds. But they still work on a business model, meaning that they have to make more than they spend. To avoid taxation, they often list the excess as "funds available for future expansion of facilities" rather than as profits.

Institutions charge for their services and try to maximize their incomes. They pay their top administrative officers large salaries (half to one-and-a-half million dollars yearly is not unusual), and the leaders set up the facility so as to make money. By using usual business methods and maximizing the payments from various insurance providers and government agencies, they increase the institution's income. The charges bear no relation to costs; charging $1.00 to $5.00 for a Tylenol capsule is common. In addition, the institutions encourage the physicians they employ to give more treatments and perform more tests and discourage them from stopping treatments. These suggestions are subtle and difficult to pin down as interfering with medical practice, but it has been reported that some hospitals' administrators have sent out memos like "Dear Doctor: We have noted that you are not using our new, state-of-the-art machine. We encourage you to use this equipment more often." Through such memos and by creating an environment where doing more is valued, they let the doctors know that their practice is being watched. Doctors are urged to conduct extra testing and treatments to bring more money into the system. In some institutions, the doctor's salary is linked to her billing.

A colleague told me about a physician he knows who described his predicament when he worked as an obstetrician and gynecologist at a hospital in Wyoming. He was called into the office of the head of the hospital and told that he would have to take a salary cut of 25 percent because "he was not doing enough hysterectomies, and the hospital was losing money." The doctor tried to explain that what he was doing was medically appropriate, but the chief rejected his explanation. The doctor took the cut in salary and left that hospital soon thereafter.

Medical programs on TV give good medical advice, but they also encourage more testing and emphasize the use of drugs that may not really be necessary for the treatment of particular diseases. Again, it is hard to say when they cross the line, but the atmosphere created is one of "Do more; it is a good thing."

ICUs also bring in extra revenue for hospitals. Personally, I do not know of hospitals putting patients into ICUs just for the money. Such cases may be relatively rare, but many other hospitals are not selective about whom they transfer to the ICU. Patients are often transferred to intensive care because they are "unstable" or very sick, regardless of whether the ICU treatment will help them.

There is a growing movement to consider the idea of "too sick for the ICU."[26] If patients are so ill that they would not benefit from the ICU, they should be given comfort care in a regular hospital bed. This is a good policy that is not adhered to often enough.

Again, remember that doctors are more likely to over-treat than under-treat, outside the ICU or in it.

When dealing with the family that wants to continue unhelpful treatments, the overall atmosphere in hospitals is such that doctors are discouraged from overriding the family's wishes, even though certain medical treatments would be unjustified and futile. No administrators tell the doctors explicitly what to do, but the institutional environment is such that they yield to the family's irrational, unjustified request to continue intensive treatments. A related attitude by hospitals is their reluctance to emphasize care and compassion. Most often, the medical providers themselves are compassionate and caring. They try to keep the patients comfortable. The administration, however, likes to project the image that their hospital provides the latest and best treatments and cures. Thus, activities that focus on comfort care are given low priority. Administrators do not want to appear to be "giving up" on patients.

In the 1990s, as I entered my sixties, I became increasingly concerned about something that had bothered me for some years. I had been conscious that many patients were being given active treatments that had no chance of helping them; what they needed was comfort care. I felt helpless in general because I did not have a say in what other doctors did; I had no control over them. But I did try my best to convince the patients for whom I was responsible to forego futile treatments and opt for comfort before they died.

By 1994 I felt I needed to do more to reduce futile treatments that cause discomfort but do not help. I thought of different ways to pass the message on to my colleagues and to those in the administration of the medical school and the hospital where I worked. I wrote articles and circulated them among my colleagues. I gave talks as part of the hospital's multiple teaching activities. The common response and reaction was "I agree with you, but what can I do?"

I created a questionnaire and distributed it to a large part of the hospital's medical providers. Over 80 percent agreed that there were frequent situations in which futile medical treatments were given when comfort care would have been better for the patients. After getting the support of my peers, I drafted a "Medical Futility Policy" and submitted it to the hospital's and medical center's administration. The head of the administration said this was a good initiative and promised to circulate it to all the doctors in the system.

To date, no policy has been formulated. The matter remains pending.

The failure of institutions to address the issue of medical futility reveals an interesting paradox in our system. It is clear that medical care in the United States is very costly, more costly than in any other country in the developed world. But excessive treatments also bring more revenue to medical systems and doctors. As James Surowieki wrote in the *New Yorker*, "One person's 'waste' is another person's 'income'—the income of doctors, nurses, hospitals, drug companies and medical-technology makers."[27] The country may be wasting resources through unnecessary treatments and tests, but doctors, nurses, hospitals and drug and device manufacturers reap big profits because of this.

Our fee-for-service system leads to over-treatment. The payment system has created a perverse environment that is expensive to the country (Medicare) and also leads to a lot of ineffective, toxic chemotherapy. This is believed to have been driven by a lobby specifically put together to support the bills in both houses of Congress. Eighteen different institutions combined their resources to make this happen.[28]

Teneille Brown, who teaches medical ethics and law at the University of Utah, recommends several mechanisms to reduce these aggressive treatments.[29] Her recommendations largely suggest changes in Medicare's method of paying for care in general and for cancer chemotherapy in particular.

She suggests reimbursement for end-of-life conversations, reasoning that if they are paid for, doctors are more likely to find time for such conversations. As mentioned earlier, Medicare subsequently approved compensating doctors $86 for a half-hour discussion of a patient's end-of-life preferences.[30] Brown also recommends that the special status of chemotherapy payments be changed. If two drugs are equally effective, only the cheaper drug should be covered.

If chemotherapy and other procedures are performed less than 48 hours prior to the patient's death, Brown proposed that they be reimbursed at a lower rate. Of course, this may require a case-by-case review, as sometimes they may be justified. The direct financial gain from buying a drug and marking up the billing should be stopped. The profit from being a "middle man" is not tolerated in other fields of medicine.

Drug Companies and Manufacturers of Medical Devices

Almost all manufacturers of drugs and medical devices are publicly traded corporations. In our system, we accept that the heads of these companies are responsible for keeping the company running at a profit, for the benefit of shareholders. This is their fiduciary responsibility.

These corporations do research. They develop new drugs and devices that help many patients. But keeping the company profitable remains their executives' primary goal. In order to achieve this goal, they advertise their drugs in medical journals to get the attention of doctors. These advertisements inform practicing physicians of the benefits the drug may bring and also inform them of the precautions they need to take and the risks of the drug. The ads often exaggerate the benefits of drugs, especially the benefits over older, less expensive medications.

But drug companies also advertise directly to the general public. These print ads and broadcast commercials are carefully written and produced, and they induce many patients to want to take that drug and to ask their doctors for prescriptions. The doctors in turn are pressured to prescribe the drug, even though the medication the patient is currently taking is controlling symptoms just fine. The average American spends many more hours watching and reading drug ads in a year than he spends with his doctor. This form of direct-to-patient advertising is not permitted in any other developed country.

Drug companies spend billions of dollars on such advertising, and it is estimated that each one of those dollars leads to many more dollars in extra drug sales. Many experts feel that many of the prescriptions that are written because of direct advertising are not needed and lead to unnecessary use of drugs.

In addition to direct advertising to patients, drug representatives meet with doctors and promote their drugs to them. These reps do what they are supposed to do—increase drug sales. The consequence, however, is that more drugs are prescribed than are really needed. At the highest corporate levels, Pfizer, one of the largest drug companies in the world, was "threatened with prosecution for one of its subsidiaries, paying large bribes to a managed care company to give preferred status to one of Pfizer's drugs."[31] This was in 2002. "Two years later, the company was again facing prosecution for similar illegal marketing activities." In 2009 Pfizer, the parent company was detected engaging in the same lucrative but flagrantly illegal marketing practices, including "bribes to medical journals to publish articles promoting such uses and much more."

The Department of Justice imposed a fine on the company, but there were no prosecutions.

In order to make their job easier and their profits larger, drug companies, most of them big corporations, lobby our members of Congress to help relax some laws and regulations. In the first quarter of 2014, the pharmaceutical industry spent $65.4 million on congressional lobbying. The companies' profits are linked to the profits of doctors who purchase and prescribe drugs at a markup—as mentioned above, another inducement for doctors to over-prescribe.[32]

In *Bad Pharma: How Drug Companies Mislead Doctors and Harm Patients*, Ben Goldacre points out that drug companies, using a variety of techniques, induce doctors to prescribe expensive, even unnecessary, drugs in order to make bigger profits for the companies.[33] Apart from the money involved, patients suffer the side effects of the drugs and, if they are seriously ill, are deprived of the comfort they could get from services like hospice and palliative care.

After many years of research, Genentech developed Avastin, which led to some improvement in the control of certain types of cancer.[34] The company undertook clinical trials with Avastin for treatment of breast cancer that had spread to other parts of the body (Stage IV). Although the drug did lead to control in some cases, it was found to be exceptionally toxic; so the FDA withdrew its approval of Avastin for treating breast cancer.

Interestingly, Medicare continues to reimburse doctors and clinics for the use of Avastin to treat breast cancer. And that is the rub. The National Comprehensive Cancer Network (NCCN), a panel of experts that recommends which drugs are suitable for which cancers, stated in its guidelines that Avastin was appropriate for metastatic breast cancer. Medicare accepted this and therefore funds Avastin. The drug is also approved for other cancers and continues to be on the market. A significant issue of conflict of interest arose with this recommendation, because 9 of the 32 members of the NCCN panel had financial ties to Genentech.[35] Such ties lead to many distortions of our medical system.

A similar process takes place with the manufacturers of medical devices, such as artificial joints, heart pacemakers and insulin pumps. Some medical devices help patients. Without them, many patients would die or suffer. But sometimes these devices are used inappropriately because of pressure by the device companies or their advisors. Often, doctors feel obligated to use a device even though its benefit has not been proven or is questionable in a particular patient's case.

It is difficult to pinpoint individual doctors or groups regarding their conducting procedures in order to increase their income. However, in her book *Knocking on Heaven's Door*, Katy Butler has written in detail about inappropriate use of cardiac pacemakers.[36] These devices can be placed under the skin below the collarbone with wires that go into the heart. A pacemaker is a very sensitive and sophisticated device that can detect the slowing or irregularity of heartbeats. If that occurs, the pacemaker sends electrical signals to the heart until the heartbeat becomes regular. Because an irregular heartbeat or very slow heart rate can cause a person to get dizzy or faint because of the lack of blood supply to the brain, the pacemaker has helped many patients feel better and has saved lives. The problem is that many patients have slow or irregular heartbeats without experiencing any problems. The use of these devices in patients without symptoms is controversial.

Monitors and pacemakers are expensive in themselves and costly to implant because of the skill required to place them in the proper manner. Unfortunately, in at least one case, kickbacks and other incentives were given to cardiologists who placed more cardiac pacemakers. During the resulting lawsuit, some companies that had paid kickbacks pleaded "no contest" to the charges and paid a fine, but the employees and physicians involved in the fraud only got suspended sentences.

The guidelines for using the pacemakers were written by a panel of experts and based on their consensus. They recommended the pacemakers for more conditions than had been the standard practice. Of the 17 experts on the panel, 11 had financial conflicts because they were paid by the manufacturers of pacemakers. For 7 of these, the conflict was so major that they were not allowed to vote. Thus collectively, if not individually, cardiologists with special training in cardiac pacemakers (electrophysiologists) had potential financial gains in recommending or installing the devices.

Overall, the cost of placing the pacemakers and related devices reached $14 billion a year by 2003. There were attempts to reduce the excessive use of pacemakers. In the *Journal of the American Medical Association* in 2009, cardiologist Pierluigi Tricoci stated, "Experts are vulnerable to conflicts of interest," and they are "strongly influenced by industry's natural desire to introduce new products."[37]

Drugs and medical devices are profitable both to the company and to the hospital. The companies persuade doctors to use their products; then the companies make deals with hospitals, which further pressure the doctors to utilize them because they all make money.

This phenomenon of excessive use of drugs, devices and treatments in general is a part of our fee-for-service system. It is difficult to say what is excessive, but the profit motive is one more reason why doctors do too much.

For well over a century, teaching hospitals in the United States have been the pillars of medical education and also the places where the best medical care was provided. Their focus was on good care by the best doctors who were also the best teachers. They taught medical students and also provided training to new graduates, who learned by hands-on experience under close supervision of their mentors. The first of such institution was the Johns Hopkins Hospital in Baltimore. The hospital was founded in 1889; the Johns Hopkins Medical School followed four years later. One of the school's four founders, William Osler, immediately began recruiting bright young doctors for further training under his supervision. Under his influence, other medical schools and the hospitals attached to them started residency training programs. This provided the patients with the best care, while the students and trainees had the best education under the direct tutelage of great teachers and doctors. Though in general the system in the United States involved patients paying for the medical services they received, teaching hospitals kept their fees low and even provided charity care, often waiving their fees for poor patients. The focus of the faculty, who were senior physicians, was teaching students and residents to provide the best possible care for the patients—not to make the most money. Along with these roles, the staff conducted research with the goal of expanding knowledge. With a few exceptions, they did not patent the products of their research and did not make extra money from it.

There have been major changes in this ideal that teaching hospitals used to follow. In her review of Kenneth M. Ludmerer's *Let Me Heal: The Opportunity to Preserve Excellence in American Medicine,* Lara Goitein states, "Residents, with little supervision, are struggling to keep up with staggering workloads, and have little time or energy left for learning. Attending physicians, for their part, are often too occupied with their own research and clinical practices— often in labs and offices outside of the hospital—to pay much attention to the house officers."[38] Because these house officers (residents) are paid far less than physicians who have completed their residencies (a first-year resident's salary, typically subsidized by Medicare, is often equivalent to that of a beginning elementary school teacher), yet provide most of the medical care, they save the hospital significant money.

The reduced importance of education and training and the shift in priorities of the faculty of medical schools and teaching hospitals led to many changes. The institutions and the individuals became focused on ways to bring in more and more money for "them." Some took on research endeavors that were lucrative, especially if they were in collaboration with drug companies. They also adjusted their clinical practices to increase revenues. As Goitein goes on to quote Ludmerer, "They followed the money, resting content with the status quo as long as clinical revenues and their own pay continued to grow."[39]

They modified their practice patterns, for example, by promoting high-revenue subspecialty and procedural approaches to medicine. They also developed a closer relationship with pharmaceutical and biotech companies and manufacturers of medical devices. This relationship allowed them to make extra money for the institution and for themselves. Because of the new priorities, they had a greater incentive to do more treatments and to place less emphasis on the comfort of the patient.

RESEARCH

Research is essential for progress. In physics, sociology and history, as in medicine, without research there can be no improvement or progress. In medicine, a few examples are worth mentioning. If we had not done research, we would have no means to treat infections; after more than six decades of research the first antibiotics were developed. In cancer, without research we would not have understood what cancer cells do and would not have been able to treat even the cancers that we can now treat successfully. Understanding body fluids through research allows us to treat patients who are dehydrated or have kidney disease.

But all research must be done systematically, with the results re-examined on an ongoing basis. Just as important, research must be conducted honestly and should be overseen by others who are not the primary researchers. A process called "peer review" requires an evaluation of the idea of the research and the way the study is conducted; peer review also helps make sure that the conclusions drawn are reasonable and within the scope of the research results. All these steps are required to ensure that the research remains accurate and meaningful. A guiding principle of science demands that if new facts are revealed, then the whole study should be reviewed, reassessed and, if needed, changed or abandoned. One example described earlier was that of William Halsted and his radical surgery for breast cancer. Research and evaluation of the results of the surgery led to halting that brutal assault on patients, even though it took decades.

Research in medicine requires many steps and involves scientists from a large variety of fields. Understanding of the structure and function of the normal body is the first step, and it alone involves anatomists, histologists, physiologists, biochemists, biophysicists and others. There are molecular biologists who study the regulation of the growth of cells and how each type of cell interacts with other cells and with the body as a whole. They measure how the body and the cells react to day-to-day stresses, exercise, sleep, dehydration and emotional challenges. Immunologists study how the body protects itself from outside chemical or biological influences. They also try to understand how the body deals with cells or tissues within the body when they "behave badly." They try to use all available tools and regularly collaborate with physicists, chemists, engineers and surface chemists. An in-depth insight into normal structure and function allows precise understanding of how the body changes when there is disease.

Those who study the body in a diseased state rely on what is known of the normal body. Like the study of the normal body, this area of medical science includes study of individual cells and their reaction to and interaction with other cells or the organ where they originate, as well as their interaction with other organs. The body works as a whole, and the relationship of a part to the whole is very important.

Among those who study the body in disease are specialists called pathologists. Pathologists are a part of the team that makes the diagnosis of a disease by examining the tissue or organ that is removed from the body in a biopsy. Usually a small amount of tissue is removed for the purpose of finding out what type of disease afflicts the organ. Pathologists also examine the whole organ or diseased area removed by the surgeon if it is not functioning well or is causing difficulty for the patient. This is a role the pathologist plays in diagnosis and is a part of the full evaluation of the patient's problem.

In addition, pathologists and others carry out research that may involve cells grown in plastic containers that are subjected to different conditions and environments. They also study disease in a variety of animals.

All the above-described research, done outside the human body, is broadly referred to as "pre-clinical." The information resulting from pre-clinical research forms the basis of research on humans, for example, involving a new drug that has properties that biomedical scientists think may be helpful in controlling a condition such as high blood pressure or diabetes. Before being tested in people, the drug is tested in animals to get information on its side effects and a general idea of the dose that would be effective and reasonably well tolerated by humans.

After this pre-clinical information is put together, the new drug is tested in human beings who volunteer to take it. These people are fully informed, verbally and in writing, and understand that there are risks involved. They are also told that the new drug may or may not work for them. The researchers monitor the subjects to see how they are responding.

Developing a new drug is a slow, carefully planned and meticulous process. It is also expensive. Understanding how a drug is developed, tested and finally available for use in patients may help you decide whether or not you would like to participate in a clinical trial if one is suggested to you by your doctor. It will also help you decide whether you are participating in the clinical trial to help other patients in the future or you are doing this with the hope of getting benefit for yourself. This is especially important when you have a difficult-to-treat disease or a disease that has not responded to previous treatments, such as advanced cancer.

The process of drug development begins with the laboratory researchers and chemists who look at defects in the abnormal cell or organ that can be (potentially) corrected by a new drug that acts on some part of the cell. This is a very specialized field and involves various types of scientists like molecular biologists, chemists, electrophysicists, etc. On the basis of their knowledge and with consensus, they decide on a chemical compound which they deduce *might* have beneficial effects. They first test their idea in the laboratory using tools appropriate for the organ or disease. They may also use small animals such as mice to do the initial testing. If they get results that suggest the drug may be worth testing further, they test it on larger animals like dogs or monkeys. If the tests in large animals confirm the original hypothesis and the drug is not too toxic, they test it in humans.

This is an important step, because research on humans has to be done very carefully. The goal is to test a new drug in a way that the risks to the people who participate are minimized and the subjects are fully informed about the trial. They need to understand what is known about the drug, what the potential benefits are and what the known harmful effects of the drug are.

This research on humans is conducted with care in order to protect the subjects while the new drug is being tested. The whole drug trial process is supervised by a board of medical and non-medical people. Some members of this board are from within the institution where the research is conducted, and some are from the community. Their role is to make sure that the person taking the new drug is fully informed about its risks. The researchers provide regular reports to this body, commonly called the Human Research Review Committee (HRRC), about how the volunteers fare during the research.

The HRRC and the research process as a whole are regulated by the FDA, the Office of Human Research Protections (OHRP) and the Department of Health and Human Services (HHS) of the federal government. This oversight has two purposes. First, it makes sure that the research is performed properly and safely. Second, it makes sure that participants are fully informed about the risks and benefits of taking part in the clinical trials. The trials are conducted in stages or "phases" in an orderly, step-by-step manner. I have been on the HRRC of our institution since 1996 and have seen many improvements in the process.

Phase I trials are performed as a first step. Only a small number of patients are included in these trials. They must be patients who have no better options for the treatment of their disease. The patients are informed clearly that the drug being tested has not been given to humans before and that there could be many harmful side effects. Also, they are informed that there may or may not be any benefit to them. Phase I trials require special expertise, so only a few selected centers are allowed to conduct them.

Once Phase I of the clinical research is completed, the results are analyzed. This analysis provides the researchers with better information about the pharmacology of the drug, such as the dosage that would be most appropriate and what kind of toxic effects the drug may cause. Based on the results, the drug goes into Phase II.

If patients with a particular disease showed some response during the Phase I trial, the study is extended to examine the efficacy of the drug in that disease. These Phase II trials are conducted on a few more patients. This allows confirmation of the information on the toxicity of the drug and makes it possible to determine the best dosage. The same strict standards for safety and patient information as Phase I are followed.

If the drug shows promise after completion of Phase II of the testing, it now is ready to be compared to previously available treatments. This is called Phase III, and the new drug is tested in a larger number of patients to be sure that the data are reliable. (If only 100 people participated in the study of a cholesterol-lowering medication, their improvement might more likely be attributable to chance than if 10,000 participated.) Again, the clinical trials are strictly regulated, monitored and subject to oversight by different committees and regulators as with Phase I and II trials. Phase III trials are usually conducted in multiple clinical trial centers so that data are generated more quickly.

The goal of Phase III is to find out if the drug is more or less efficacious and more or less toxic than previously available drugs. In order to do this, and to avoid bias, the patients are randomized to receive the new drug or the standard drug. This means that patients 1, 3, 5, 7, etc., receive the new drug and patients 2, 4, 6, 8, etc., receive the standard drug. Sometimes this sorting is done with a computer to eliminate bias further. (If the new drug treats a relatively minor condition, for example, teenage acne, for which the volunteers are not currently taking medication, half the participants usually receive a placebo—a "sugar pill.")

If the new drug is more effective or less toxic than the previously available drug, the information is sent to the FDA. The FDA independently evaluates the data, and they decide if the new drug should be approved for general use.

Even after a new drug is approved for clinical use, in the early months and years the drug is monitored by the FDA. This provides an added measure of safety. This monitoring is sometimes called Phase IV clinical research, but it is often used as a marketing tool.

Thus, in summary, new drugs and treatments are supposed to be developed systematically and carefully under close scrutiny. However, drug company funding of the research may influence results.

From your perspective as a patient, what you need to consider is: Should I participate in a clinical trial? Some doctors will suggest that you participate in a clinical trial to avoid giving you bad news. They use the hope raised by clinical trials to escape from dealing with death and may delay the comfort measures that could give you a better end of life.

All clinical trials are conducted primarily to generate data that will help scientists develop new drugs or other treatments. Your participation in the research may help future patients, because, partly thanks to you, doctors will learn more about the disease and what works and what does not. Maybe this will make you feel good—if not physically, then emotionally; maybe it will provide a positive outlet for your anger at your disease. Participation in research to help others is laudable. But if your reason for taking part in research is the hope of a benefit for yourself, make sure you get detailed information from your doctor about what this might realistically be.

The chances of benefit to you personally vary with the phase of the trial and the nature of your disease, but do not make the all-too-common mistake of assuming that a clinical trial is a chance to receive a "miracle cure" that will make you live longer or feel better than the medication you are currently taking. You should read the information about the study carefully and discuss it with your friends and family. Think about it. Ask questions about the trial. Talk both to your own doctor and to the doctor conducting the trial. Only then should you decide whether to participate. Do it for yourself, or do it to help future patients, but be informed and thus empowered.

Other types of research on humans consist of systematic analysis of data on populations of patients and healthy people (epidemiological research). This type of research can lead to identification of factors that predict disease or identify risk factors for disease—what food or drink is better to maintain health, or what effect obesity and activity have on health and longevity. For example, epidemiological research confirmed that cigarette smoking causes cancer.

Thus, many types of research are being performed in medicine. All ages, people at risk for or afflicted with all diseases and all demographic groups have benefited. Not just better understanding of the body (normal and abnormal) but new techniques and drugs have been the result of the research that has been conducted on humans over a long period of time.

However, a number of problems exist with the research system in the United States. These are briefly summarized here to provide an understanding of why there is success and why there are failures—why certain diseases are still not fully understood or why they cannot be treated. There are also inherent limitations as to what can ultimately be achieved, and there are limitations or problems because of how the research is conducted.

Bioethicist Daniel Callahan, co-founder of the Hastings Center near New York City, has studied and written extensively on the subject.[40] His main point is that research in the field of medicine and medical care has been focused on prolonging life and finding cures for specific diseases. This is not to negate the research that led to the control of infectious diseases and epidemics that had a major impact on the quality of life and longevity of humans throughout the world. For example, tuberculosis and gastrointestinal infections, the second and third causes of death in 1900, did not even appear among the top 15 in 2010.[41] The benefits of good nutrition, hygiene, clean water and immunization are obvious and unquestioned. These advances took place more than a hundred years ago, and the development of antibiotics, beginning in the 1940s, changed a lot of lives. Here the control of bacteria-caused diseases and infections from wounds led directly to a better and longer life for millions of people. Improvement in the care of mothers and newborns has also had a major impact on the health of the population. Unfortunately, the United States lags behind other developed countries in this field.

More recently, our emphasis has changed, and we are now paying more attention, spending more money and putting a lot more effort into understanding specific diseases and also into increasing longevity. We have become focused on thinking of death and disease as the ultimate enemy. This is well and good within limits, but by trying to eliminate all disease and death, we have ignored the person. Research that is driven by funding priorities, encouraged by advocacy groups and targeted at eliminating *all* disease and increasing lifespan has caused many problems. The false hope generated by such advocacy has, in a sense, left the person behind.

The need now is to implement the benefits of the knowledge we have. We know that smoking and obesity cause many serious problems; they affect the quality of life of millions and shorten the lives of many. People suffer and die early because we have not made enough effort to implement what we have already learned. Callahan advises us to work on reducing premature deaths, reducing disability and stressing comfort at the time of death. We should not try to eliminate all diseases and should not try to live forever.[42] One area of research that lags behind is why, despite the evidence, obesity and smoking rates remain high.

In the sixties, speakers at high school graduations inspired the students with stories of astronauts and space scientists. Those professions were considered to be the ultimate achievement for young people going out into the world. Nowadays, cancer research, finding a cure for cancer, is considered to be the height of achievement. At my granddaughter's graduation the keynote speaker on three occasions stated, "Even if you don't find the cure for cancer, you can still do great things." As Callahan says, this sends the wrong message about research priorities. For example, social science research on how to help patients and families cope with the consequence of illness is sadly neglected.

Late in 2015, a book by Vincent T. DeVita Jr., *The Death of Cancer*, appeared to considerable fanfare.[43] DeVita directed the National Cancer Institute from 1980 to 1988 and spearheaded the development of revolutionary new treatments for Hodgkin's disease, a cancer of the lymph glands. The treatments developed by DeVita and his colleagues resulted in cures for a disease that had previously meant almost certain death. They also opened up important avenues for new and effective treatments for many other cancers.

The Death of Cancer is a personal memoir and a clear and compelling history of the development of chemotherapy and medical oncology. The credit for this progress belongs in large part to DeVita, for his hard work, his leadership and his passion. In fact, many in the field have called him "St. Vincent." But DeVita is also a proselytizer and a true believer. He seems not to understand, or at least not to accept, the law of diminishing returns. He pioneered a treatment for a fatal disease when there was no other treatment. He led the National Cancer Institute during a crucial period of its development and was a major force in the creation of the "War on Cancer" a few years later. He now states that cancer could be cured if the doctors were bold enough and the FDA did not stifle innovation. DeVita uses positive anecdotes and his own success to make his point.

However, he also employs selective statistics without putting them in context to make the case that cancer therapy has been a success. This distinguished and influential researcher neglects to explain that only a small number of cancers have been cured.

DeVita describes many of the conflicts he had with Congress and numerous government agencies and relates how he was able to prevail. His simplistic, even evangelical, ideas are similar to those of many other oncologists. This is good—to a point. Government funding and political support are essential to research. But this mind-set becomes destructive when it raises unrealistic expectations in the public, and especially in patients and their families—when it creates false hope.

Despite what Congress and government agencies like the National Institutes of Health may do, the main drivers of biomedical research, the big sources of funding and the disbursement of publicity, are advocacy groups and drug companies. Large amounts of money and publicity (which leads to funding by the government) are generated by one or another advocacy group for specific diseases. This practice is fine to a point, but it directs attention piecemeal to certain diseases without taking into account the commonness of the disease or how much and how it affects people. For example, when the world loses renowned actors and artists to a disease such as AIDS, public attention and funding follow. Thanks to the resulting accelerated research, medical science developed drugs that have transformed HIV/AIDS into a chronic disease, rather than the death sentence it was originally. But in the meantime, researchers focusing on diseases that primarily afflict the poor have had their funding cut, and campaigns to prevent birth defects and chronic diseases receive little notice. The priorities are skewed.

The other big problem is bias in conducting the research. Bias starts with the conduct of clinical trials that drug companies sponsor and fund. The funding of biomedical research has changed significantly in recent years. It is now a $100 billion enterprise. Support from pharmaceutical companies increased from 32 percent in 1980 to 62 percent in 2003.[44]

Even though clinical trials are regulated by government bodies, the drug companies can find loopholes. They withhold publication of data from trials that did not support their drugs. They manipulate—not necessarily falsify—the results. They use statistical tricks to make small differences look big. They use words like "may," "could" and "promising" to promote the use of their drugs. According to a report in the *Journal of the American Medical Association*, "Research results published by pharmaceutical industry-sponsored investigators are far more likely to have outcomes favoring the sponsor than research funded by other sources."[45]

The system as a whole employs hype, exaggerations and publicity to increase research grants and donations. Even non-profit organizations, like university medical centers, use research to induce patients to come to their centers, because it means more revenue. Early in 2014, I received a brochure from Yale University's Cancer Center. It described the work they are doing—which is laudable. What bothered me was this statement: "That's where clinical trials come into cancer medicine. . . . They offer the hope that patients and providers want."[46]

By its nature a clinical trial is testing, trying to find out if a drug works. This is especially true of Phase I and Phase II trials where very new and poorly understood drugs are being tested. To say that clinical trials offer "hope" is an overstatement. They offer hope to future patients but not to the ones who participate in the trials.

In addition, there have been instances of misuse and misconduct in research. This does not and should not lead to discontinuing research; nor does it mean that as patients we should stop participating in research. It does mean that when asked to participate in clinical trials, we should ask questions and be reassured that a particular trial is right for us.

Misconduct in research has occurred at some of the best known and respected institutions, as well as some smaller but recognized medical centers and universities. Johns Hopkins Medical School,[47] University of Washington Medical Center[48] and University of Pennsylvania[49] are among the offenders. Proper oversight by federal agencies led to correction of some of these problems. The common threads in these instances of misconduct were the researchers' unquestioning and unquestioned belief in the idea that they were testing. The idea was certainly a good one based on the science and the animal experiments they had conducted on that particular disease. Having pioneering ideas is a sign of brilliance. Unfortunately, many smart people are also ambitious. Due to their ambition, their confidence and their faith in their own intelligence, these scientists did not follow the rules. They took shortcuts and conducted research on humans before they had fully studied the effect of their idea in animals. This resulted in tragedies, including deaths of some patients and even of a healthy young woman volunteer. Regulatory bodies have become more strict and vigilant, and misconduct in research has been reduced. However, there is potential gain to the investigators who conduct the research. Fame and fortune may result, so they may cut corners.

In some cases, there is potential financial gain either for the researchers or for the institutions they are affiliated with. This clouds their judgment. By federal regulation, investigators must disclose any financial interest they have to the appropriate authorities *and* to the patient considering participation in the research. Most researchers believe that the research they are conducting will lead to progress in the understanding or treatment of the disease the patient is suffering from. Their motive is appropriate and worthy. But some become over-ambitious and may misrepresent the nature of the research. They may overstate the benefits of the treatment they are testing, or they may underplay the risk of side effects, maybe without malice but because of hope. But misconduct does occur.

One recent problem was revealed in an editorial in the *New York Times* about psychiatric research at the University of Minnesota.[50] Abuses ranged from one psychiatrist participating despite a suspended license to another enrolling Hmong refugees, who were illiterate and thus unable to give informed consent. The author charged that the problem was not confined to the Department of Psychiatry but extended to the university administration: "Rather than dealing forthrightly with these ethical abuses, university officials have seemed more interested in covering up wrongdoing with a variety of underhanded tactics."

Not all research is of the same quality. Some may not provide any significant improvement in the understanding or treatment of a disease. In academic institutions, all professors and trainees are required to do some form of research. Sometimes, a study is undertaken just to satisfy the requirements of the institution. If the researcher is not really versed in the topic and does not have good ideas, the research has no meaning and may not benefit anyone. But in order to satisfy the conditions of his or her job, the researcher may try to persuade you to participate in the study.

Research, when properly conducted on the appropriate patient is the best, in fact the only, way to achieve progress in medicine. In some cases, a study may offer the patient a chance to receive a treatment not otherwise available. Patients should participate in research where appropriate, but only after understanding the full nature of their disease and the details of the research.

Remember, some doctors will suggest that you participate in a clinical trial to avoid giving you bad news. They use the hope raised by clinical trials to escape from dealing with death and may delay the comfort measures that could give you a better end of life.

10

Why Doctors Over-Treat

Flaws in the Way They Deal with Patients

Dealing with very sick patients is emotionally challenging. Doctors deal with this in many different ways. Some are related to their belief systems, while others are related in the way they react to a patient's stated wish. These reasons include the following:

a. Hope, "just in case"
b. Belief in technology
c. Going along with the patient's wishes
d. Fear of death
e. Desire to be thorough and complete
f. Incompetence
g. Failure to address religious and spiritual needs

HOPE, "JUST IN CASE"

Some doctors are so reluctant to stop treatment that they will try unproven, even ineffective treatments. They say, "There may be some hope," or recommend a treatment "just in case" it works. This is how some doctors deal with perceived failure. What the patient needs is hope for comfort and assurance of honest communication, not false hope for a cure or substantial remission. But the doctor who over-treats usually ends up hurting you. They also hurt the people working with them; junior colleagues are obliged to follow the orders of the "senior" doctor. Following orders for a futile, painful treatment is morally distressing, but the junior doctors and the nursing staff are required to do so.

However, this is not an easy decision. I would like to quote from a blog sent by Thaddeus Pope, a medical ethicist who is a lawyer by training:

> In preparing for a talk in Michigan this week, I was refreshing myself on some of the key health care decisions laws from that state. One of the most significant is the Supreme Court's 1995 decision in In re Martin. I love this quote:
>
> The decision to accept or reject life-sustaining treatment has no equal. We enter this arena humbly acknowledging that neither law, medicine nor philosophy can provide a wholly satisfactory answer to this question.
>
> To err **either way** has incalculable ramifications. To end the life of a patient who still derives meaning and enjoyment from life or to condemn persons to lives from which they cry out for release is nothing short of barbaric. If we are to err, however, we must err in preserving life.
>
> Many judges have made similar observations about balancing errors of unwanted death against errors of unwanted life. Perhaps the most famous was by Justice Brennan in Cruzan.
>
> **But must the resolution of this tension always be to err in favor of life? Mountains of evidence indicates that errors of unwanted life swamp errors of unwanted death by exponential proportions. How many must suffer to mitigate the chance that one might die too soon? We have surely long surpassed that number.**[1]

The judge whom Pope quoted, the late Justice William Brennan, was in the minority in the 1989 case of *Cruzan v Director, Missouri Department of Health*, in which the United States Supreme Court ruled five-to-four that the family of a 29-year-old woman rendered permanently unconscious six years earlier by an automobile accident had no right to have her taken off life support. The ruling was overturned six months later after the Cruzans were able to provide further evidence that their daughter did not want to continue life in what doctors call "a persistent vegetative state."[2]

To put Justice Brennan's eloquent words into simple English is not easy without losing their full significance. What I get out of them is that we tend to err on the side of doing more, just in case our treatment works. But, he asks, is that the correct approach?

Sometimes false hope on the part of the doctors matches up with your false hope as the patient. As a result, you may subject yourself to futile, ineffective, treatments, and this delays implementation of comfort measures that would lead to a good death.

"Just in case" is fine when you look both ways even if you have a green light—it costs nothing and averts an injury if there happens to be some impaired driver about to run a red light. "Just in case" is not appropriate when someone is dying. Honesty, communication and empathy are what are needed.

With the advances in medical knowledge and treatments, there are many diseases that can now be successfully treated. The success of these advances is not universal. Some patients respond to the treatment, and others do not. There is often more than one treatment available for the same disease. The success rate of the different treatments is generally known. Logically, the first treatment that is tried is the one with the best known results. If this does not work, then the next best treatment is tried and so on.

As an example, suppose the first treatment is successful in 70 percent of patients. Doctors will try that one first. If the treatment does not work or the disease returns after initial control, then they will try the second-best treatment. (The terms often used are "first line," "second line," etc.) Say the success of the second line treatment is 30 percent. It would seem reasonable to try that treatment. However, as we go down the line, the situation changes. The third line treatment may work in 15 percent of cases, and the fourth line may be effective for a short time in 5 percent of situations.

To decide if the first line treatment is worthwhile is easy; most people would try it. Probably the same would be true for second line treatments. But the benefits of third and fourth line treatments are small, and it is important to think about each carefully. Is it worthwhile? Are the small benefit and chance of response to treatment worth the side effects and your precious time? This should be your decision, but you should make it only after due consideration and seeing if trying these additional treatments fits with your values and goals.

I had a patient from a small town in New Mexico. She was 18 years old, beautiful, smart and sensible. So was her husband. She had a familial type of breast cancer, and many of her cousins and aunts currently had or had had this cancer. The initial treatment was successful, and the young woman enjoyed a good quality of life for 10 years. When she was in her late twenties, the cancer recurred, and the next treatment also worked—for a few months. At that time, we discussed the problem, and I consulted my colleagues. They said, "Yes, there are other treatments, but they have a small chance of working. The tumor may shrink, but it will be for a short time."

By this point, the cancer had spread to many parts of my patient's body, and she was in pain. After due discussion, we all agreed that further chemotherapy would only increase her problems. With a heavy heart, she went home to die in peace in the comfort of her family. It was hard on me.

The outcome was sad, but it would have been sadder if she had undergone more treatments.

As discussed above, there are many reasons why doctors do too much, most of them with good intentions. However, you as the patient must agree with the recommendations and actions proposed by the doctor before you accept the treatment. Ask questions, feel comfortable about what is in *your* best interest, and only then consent to, or reject, the treatment.

BELIEF IN TECHNOLOGY

Recently, I was talking to a friend who is a physicist. He got his PhD from Harvard and works at a major national laboratory. We started discussing choices at the end of life. He began by telling me he was not sure what he would want for himself. Soon, he started saying technology *could do* so much. "There is so much research and progress that I would like to take advantage of all that," he told me. He is smart, accomplished, 56 years old and in good health. However, he does not understand biology too well and is unaware of the limitations of medical technology and what can be realistically achieved. He was unable to make a distinction between what *can* be done now and what *may* be possible in the future. This optimism is understandable, especially from a physicist who has seen remarkable progress in his own field leading to greater understanding of the mysteries of the universe.

Doctors also are scientists and are trained to look at the information, to analyze it and to make decisions based on their evaluation of the same. This is the basis of their recommendations to their patients. Most often they do it well. But they also may develop too much faith in technology. They have, after all, seen progress in medical science made over the years: new understanding of diseases, new technology for diagnosis, better outcomes from surgery, and new effective drugs. Therefore, they are optimistic regarding further progress in the future. In their enthusiasm, in their optimism, they forget the law of diminishing returns. They forget that progress is incremental and that with each step the increment is smaller. The first steps are easier, but it gets more difficult to get similar advances with later steps.

What does that mean to you as a patient? Every time doctors are faced with a situation where a patient does not respond to a treatment, they look for other forms of treatment. They look for the research reports or ideas that have been written about in journals. They think of ways to improve on what they have tried. They are looking out for you.

The problem arises when their belief in technology clouds their judgment. They may not put the reported "advance" into perspective. They may get inappropriately enthusiastic about it. The advance may be in a disease or situation not exactly like yours. They still suggest trying the new treatment. You may or may not receive the full explanation of the treatment and its applicability to your case. If all the right questions are not asked, you may make a decision that is not fully informed. The doctors' faith in technology and their focus on the disease may lead to the use of treatments based on hope rather than reason. Also, the science behind the new treatments can be very interesting and tantalizing; it stimulates their minds; they want to see it in action. Hope, as we all know, is important. But when deciding on approaches to difficult-to-treat diseases, reason is more important. Jerome Groopman has put it well: "Our technology had advanced but our thinking has not kept pace."[3] Advances in medical science and technology have accomplished a lot. However, when they lead to doing too much, they complicate the end of life rather than improving it.

Biology is different from physics. The living body is much more complex than subatomic particles. A lot has been accomplished in biology. In the laboratory, we have developed understanding of the genes, the enzymes and the chemical reactions that control the stability and growth of cells. We now know a lot about cancer cells and how they differ from normal cells. By understanding that cancer cells need more of certain nutrients, it was possible to develop drugs that starved the cancer cells and caused them to die. By understanding the enzymes that do not work normally in cancer cells, it was possible to regulate them and make them behave more like normal cells. Many of these discoveries have been translated into successful treatments of cancer in animals. Some of them have controlled cancer in humans. But it takes an increasing amount of research, and more complicated research, to understand each part of the cell. Even greater effort is required to apply that knowledge to humans, and enormous amounts of further effort, time and money will be necessary to develop another successful treatment of even one type of cancer. With each advance in knowledge, the complexity of the problem increases, and the new scientific insight may or may not lead to an effective treatment.

To give another example: it took decades of research to show that cholesterol causes the hardening of the arteries (atherosclerosis) that leads to heart attacks and stroke. Even after more decades of research, it is not clear how and why cholesterol gets deposited in the arteries. There have been significant advances in the treatment of atherosclerosis, as there have been in the treatment of different types of cancer. But each step takes more effort and results in fewer advances in treatment; the law of diminishing returns is at work. As knowledge increases, the problem becomes more complex. Each further advance requires more and more effort and money, and many studies, even the best-run, yield no applicable results.

Medical researchers have been working to improve the health of people for centuries. As mentioned previously, clean water and safe food accomplished a lot. Antibiotics and vaccines controlled many infectious diseases. But now we are dealing with more complexities, each needing more and more research and understanding, more work and time and, yes, more and more money—money that could be used to solve many problems in the world. It does not make sense to expect technology to fix all our problems.

My physicist friend's hope that biomedical science *may* accomplish a lot is fine. We must, however, be realistic and understand that there are limits to what medicine can do. As I noted earlier, Hasting Institute bioethicist Daniel Callahan has pointed out that it is unreasonable to expect that we can eliminate all diseases. Certainly, we cannot eliminate death. He suggests that we should concentrate our efforts on making it easier to deal with disease and death rather than trying to eliminate them.[4] If we conducted research to find out why people continue to smoke, continue to eat unhealthy foods and don't take care of themselves, we could help a lot of people lead better, longer lives and enjoy their lives until they die.

GOING ALONG WITH THE PATIENT'S WISHES
Often patients, in their desperation, ask the doctor to "do something" and "not give up." This is understandable. But it is in your best interest as a patient

that you undergo only reasonable and potentially effective treatments, as confirmed by medical knowledge and experience. The doctor should inform you of the limits of what can and cannot be done, even if giving you this information involves a difficult conversation. If appropriate, she should say that there are no treatments available. But doctors, at times, just go along with the patient's request and agree to try a treatment that you *both know* is not going to work and may even cause harm. Rather than give in to this impulse, the doctor should explain the situation. This requires confidence, understanding, compassion and time, and many physicians, for a variety of reasons, are unable to have this talk.

On the other hand, I had a patient with metastatic breast cancer. She and her husband were both bright, active, intelligent people. She had had breast cancer several years earlier. This time, she presented with abdominal pain and had a rare manifestation of metastatic deposits in her pancreas and on the lining of her lungs. Choice of chemotherapy was difficult because at the time of the original diagnosis, she had already received chemotherapy, an example of the first-line treatment explained above. We were able to give her additional chemotherapy with a drug she had not had earlier. After two rounds of this, the tumors shrank, and she felt better. However, when her symptoms returned and the tumor was once again growing, she wanted to try more treatments.

At the time of our conversation, the patient was somewhat weaker, but still was active and enjoying her family and friends. On consulting the literature, I did find some drugs that had, according to some articles, resulted in some shrinkage of tumors in patients in her situation. I discussed the options with her and her husband. I explained the reality—yes, there were treatments available, but the benefit was small and for a short time. After deliberating, they decided not to take further treatment and instead chose comfort care with the help of hospice. My patient died comfortably at home about three months later.

A few months after my patient's death, I ran into her husband at an Easter concert. He was sad but was doing all right and carrying on his life. He thanked me for the care I had given and for the time they could share while his wife was under hospice care. Explaining the situation had allowed them to accept the reality and enjoy a good quality of life in her last months.

Just following a patient's request for an ineffective treatment may seem like the easiest course, but it is not in the patient's best interest. Doing more in these cases is not helpful to the patient, but doctors give in to this impulse commonly.

FEAR OF DEATH

Like all of us, doctors have a fear of death. One way they attempt to combat that fear is by doing too much. They try treatments just to avoid dealing with death. But that is not helpful and causes more pain to the patient. Death will occur in spite of the doctor's treatments, because of the nature of the disease.

As I explained earlier, some doctors also are unable to give bad news. They avoid telling patients that the treatment has failed. I have a friend who is knowledgeable and also very kind, but he has had a hard time telling patients that the treatments they have received have not controlled their disease. He relies on other people to give the bad news. He uses euphemisms like "Things don't look good," when what he needs to say is "We have tried our best to treat the disease, and nothing has succeeded. Keeping you comfortable should be our goal now. We will go through this together." Since it is so hard for him to say these words, he goes ahead and suggests another treatment despite his understanding that it will not help. On several occasions, he has admitted patients to the hospital for more treatments even though the patients' cancers had progressed despite previous treatments and the patients were very weak. I had the responsibility of managing the treatment of my friend's patients when they were hospitalized. I was not comfortable giving chemotherapy to these patients, who were weak and frail, so I called my friend and asked if I could discuss hospice with the patient. He said, "Sure, go ahead." The point is that he could not talk about hospice but was happy to have someone else do it.

The medical system in general reinforces the fear of death. Our professional culture considers death to be the ultimate enemy. With that attitude, we transfer our own fear of death to our patients. The doctors' fear and the patient's fear reinforce each other. The result is over-treatment when comfort care and a good death would benefit all concerned.

Here is a quote from a medical student who had been an EMT before entering medical school. These are Quinn Bailey's own words:

Most recently, a patient who was treated by my team in internal medicine was hospitalized with lung disease, which progressed rapidly. He was discharged with the possibility of being placed on hospice. His husband called to let our team know that he died a day after discharge. He also expressed gratitude for the care his husband had received. I was glad for him, that he was able to die at home, among loved ones. I was also happy that those involved in his care had done all in their power not just to treat his illness, but to help him and those he loved make the transition easier, as he neared death. At this point in my life, I tend to view death with minimal discomfort. After having seen a great deal of death, I can view it with acceptance and serenity. It is an [in]evitable outcome—and integral part—of life.

DESIRE TO BE THOROUGH AND COMPLETE

Thoroughness is an essential part of a doctor's training. Physicians are taught to take a detailed history, examine the patient from head to toe and conduct the needed tests. On the basis of this information, and what the patient tells them, they develop a list of causes that could explain the patient's problems. They list the problems, match them with other information and create a priority list—meaning what is more or less likely to explain what is happening to the patient. Sometimes diagnosis is easy—a patient falls, has an injury to the hand, and the X-ray shows a broken bone. Her doctors know what to do. In some cases, the problem is more complex and requires further thinking and testing. They continue to do what is needed to gather relevant information until they have an answer and can work out a treatment plan.

There is another way things may proceed. After the initial history and examination, the doctor can create a list of differential diagnoses, a list of conditions that may explain in some way what the patient has. The list may include, say, six possible causes of the patient's problem. Some doctors may decide that of these six, only one is relevant and likely in that patient. They work with that diagnosis, make a plan and implement it. Other physicians may decide they need to be sure whether any of the others apply to the patient, so they do further testing to "rule in" or "rule out" the other five.

A friend of mine who is in excellent health at age 75 worked in his yard all day on a hot day. By his own admission, he did not drink adequately. That evening when he got up from the toilet, he felt dizzy, fell and hit his head on the bathroom door. He remained fully conscious, and the injury was minor. His wife took him to the urgent care center. They found nothing but a mild decrease in blood pressure, and blood tests showed that he was dehydrated.

After a few hours of fluids, he was well and went home. However, the doctors ordered a CT scan of the head and tests on his heart. Why!? They wanted to make sure he did not have a skull fracture or bleeding into his brain. Even though the injury was mild and he had no signs of bleeding, they ordered these tests because they wanted to rule out internal bleeding.

But why the heart tests!? Because the list also includes heart disease as a cause of dizziness. Were they being thorough, or were they doing too much? There is no absolute answer, but I think they did too much.

Doctors do too much for a variety of reasons. Deciding if a test they recommend is too much or not can be difficult. But you should ask your doctor a few simple questions: Will this test add to what we already know about me or my disease? Will the new information change the treatment or the outcome? There is no harm in asking.

The whole idea of being "thorough" has been questioned recently. The standards are being revised. As I mentioned above, many medical societies, including those for family practice, oncology and cardiology, have made a list of tests that are currently done frequently but have been shown not to be useful. The panel of experts from these societies has developed a list of things that doctors should *not* do, at least not routinely, thus reducing the number of tests conducted just for the sake of being thorough and complete. Unfortunately, this advice is not followed in many cases.

INCOMPETENCE

Some doctors do a lot of tests because they cannot figure out the patient's illness. They do "shotgun" tests hoping they will get an answer. Rather than analyzing the problem, they just order more tests. In most cases, these tests lead to no benefit and may lead to harm.

I worked with a doctor who was not very good at what he did. In one case, he demonstrated his lack of understanding of very basic medical facts. Lung cancer is difficult to treat. In some cases, if discovered early, the cancer may be removed surgically. Before undertaking surgery, it is essential that we make sure the cancer is truly small and has not spread to the adjacent parts of the body. The first test that should be conducted to show this is an X-ray of the chest. If the X-ray reveals that the cancer has spread, surgery is not worth doing. Even if the X-ray is normal, the cancer may have spread. To determine that, a competent doctor orders other, more sensitive tests if the initial X-ray shows no spread. But if the first X-ray shows a spread, no further testing is needed.

This physician saw a patient in whom the X-ray showed clear evidence of spread of the cancer. Despite that, he ordered the more sensitive tests, which obviously also showed evidence of spread. I cannot figure out why he ordered the second set of tests. To me, it demonstrated a basic lack of understanding of the process. He had many such mishaps. I understand that his senior colleagues did discuss these issues with him and tried to educate him.

Some doctors even use shotgun treatments—not just shotgun tests—because they do not understand what they should do. They just start a treatment without any thought about what they are doing. Yes, sometimes one has to treat without a full understanding of the problem. If the patient is sick, sometimes the doctors have to work on the most likely possible hypothesis, but that is after they have analyzed the problem and decided to go with the best interpretation of the data. When doctors conduct a test or recommend a treatment, they should have a reason for it, even if it is not fully clear what they are dealing with. Some doctors do too much because of incompetence and ignorance.

FAILURE TO ADDRESS RELIGIOUS AND SPIRITUAL NEEDS

Patients and families have different beliefs and needs. Some believe in a specific God or deity or force. Others are more general in their faith, and some have no concern for spirituality or afterlife. Some believe that faith can heal. Doctors have similar differences—some physicians are religious; others are not.

For a long time, it was customary in medical practice not to ask the patient or family about their religious beliefs. Discussion of religion or spirituality was not a part of the physician-patient interaction unless the patient or the family brought it up. More recently, we have accepted the idea that paying due attention to religion—whatever its nature—is helpful to both the patient and the family, and also to the medical providers. Even if there are differences in religious beliefs between the two, it is better for each party to accept and respect the other. This free communication allows appropriate religious professionals or trained persons to be brought in to provide understanding of different points of view.

In a study published in the *Journal of the American Medical Association*,[5] researchers found that those patients and families who felt that their religious or spiritual feelings were addressed, or even acknowledged, were more likely to accept the seriousness of their situation. The study was conducted on patients with metastatic cancers who were not responding to treatment and for whom the doctors had recommended comfort measures. Those who felt that their spiritual needs were paid attention to by the medical providers were more likely to accept the doctors' advice. If they felt that their belief was given due importance, they trusted the doctors more. In this study, the doctors' religious or spiritual beliefs were not taken into account. The important point was that the patients' and their families' beliefs were recognized and accepted, thus increasing their trust of the medical professionals.

As discussed in chapter 3, religion is important at times of difficulty, and paying due respect to it makes it easier for the family and the person who is dying to accept the inevitable. Death is easier and more peaceful if we acknowledge and respect religious beliefs.

In this chapter and the two preceding it, I have listed a number of reasons why doctors do too much. The motives and thinking behind doing too much vary from doctor to doctor. The main point to remember is that it is more common for doctors to do too much than too little. From your point of view as a patient, if the doctor says there is no more treatment he can offer, that is usually the case—unless you are dealing with a rare uncaring doctor. So discuss options with your doctor, but remember that it is in your best interest to accept the reality and to change your goals to comfort and togetherness with your family as the best outcome before death occurs.

Here is a poem I wrote to explain what can happen during a difficult situation:

10/14/05
What we say - What we do
It is an enigma
It is a dilemma
People seem reasonable
They seem amiable
They are thinking
They are even inking
They agree with the idea
But they fail to support

What I purport
They agree patients suffer
When we offer
Treatments that cause hurt
Treatments that don't comfort
But they still offer treatments
That only cause discomfort
Why do we offer false hope
We should give solace
Dying has a place
We all die
We should have Comfort
We should have Peace
We should have Respite

(Note: My poem offers a new meaning of CPR: comfort, peace, respite.)

11

When Doctors Say "No"

In previous chapters, I have mentioned treatments that would not help the patient because (1) the disease was too advanced for the patient to tolerate the treatment, (2) the patient had more than one problem affecting different organs, or (3) there was no treatment available with a reasonable chance of controlling the disease(s) the patient had. The terms "futile," "inappropriate" and "unreasonable" have been used when attempts are made to treat a patient in such a situation rather than to work toward the patient's comfort and care.

There are two problems with the idea of futile treatments—uncertainty and a lack of a clear definition of what is futile. Although I have brought up the issue of medical futility throughout these pages, we still have to contend with the problems of definition and uncertainty. That is because after decades of debate and numerous discussions on this topic, no consensus has been reached on appropriate definitions. Medical ethicists, physicians, lawyers and philosophers continue to debate the issue.

The first question is whether we even need to have a definition. Do we need to solve the issue of uncertainty? Can we work on the principle of *reasonable* certainty? The real issue is whether we come to a consensus on a given patient at the time of the medical crisis as to whether any treatment will make that patient better or even feel better. If we consider each patient, in his or her specific circumstance, can we say a particular treatment is futile? *In most cases, we can.* If we look at the patient's condition, the status of the disease and the treatments already tried without benefit, we can come to a consensus. If we have realistic goals, if we look at the whole picture, we can say, "This is futile," as in the case of the man with lung cancer that had spread to the brain and for whom all previous treatments did not work. Yes, the situations can be complex, but by looking at each one carefully, we can most often agree on what is futile. We have explored this before, especially in chapters 8 through 10 on why doctors over-treat. Calling treatments "futile" is just another way of saying the same thing. Long-shot treatments, given "just in case," are similar to futile treatments. If it is clear from the outset that the treatment will not help the patient, it is a futile treatment.

I have said such treatments do not help or benefit the patient. Some of my colleagues and students have raised an issue with two key words "help" and "benefit." To them these terms should be defined by the patient. These colleagues and students say that if the patient thinks it is a help or a benefit to have possibly a few weeks of additional life while continuing to endure painful symptoms, that should be considered a benefit. If having a few extra days on a ventilator is a benefit in the patient's perception, that judgment should be accepted and the treatment continued.

Others feel that the medical professionals who have the knowledge, expertise and experience should decide if a treatment should be provided or continued. We are talking about medical treatments—active interventions into the body of a person. These should be done only if, in the opinion of medically trained people, they are needed, likely to be helpful and considered proper medical practice.

(You would not have a doctor cut off someone's finger if the patient has a headache—not even if the patient considered amputation of the finger to be a benefit.)

Any treatment should result from a medical decision based on full evaluation of the patient. Yes, the family and the patient must be convinced that the given treatment is futile. The doctors must listen to their thoughts and their perception of the situation and make every effort to understand why the patient and family want to continue active treatments. For example, it would be one thing if family members explained that they wanted the patient to "hang on" for three more days so that a grown son flying in from Dubai could arrive to say goodbye. In that case, if the treatment was likely to prolong the patient's life for a week, even though the side effects would be unpleasant and the benefits would be short-lived, the doctor might agree. But if the family members said they wanted the patient to be kept alive to give medical science time to develop a "miracle cure," the doctor would need to sit down with them and explain carefully that this was a totally unrealistic approach.

The patient and family must be given a full explanation of the reasons why the treatment would be futile at that time for that patient. The responsibility of explaining the facts and the circumstances belongs to the medical professionals. If the facts are presented sympathetically and with proper explanation, most people will understand. It is best that there be consensus and agreement between the medical team and the patient and family. Stopping treatments without proper explanation can cause resentment and hostility. The process should be open and above board.

In June 2015, multiple societies involved with critical care medicine collaborated in issuing an official statement regarding disputes in ICUs. The statement focused on situations in which patients or their surrogates wanted to start or continue a treatment that the medical providers felt was not going to help the patient, was painful or wasted precious resources.[1] Classifying such disputes on the basis of the medical facts and the legal parameters that come into play in these situations, the statement analyzes the different levels of "futility" and recommends actions in each of these circumstances. The emphasis is on due process that is fair to all and on dialogue that leads to a solution that satisfies the needs of all parties. The goal is to reconcile differences and produce a result that gives appropriate weight to the judgment of the medical professionals and to the desires of the patient and surrogates.

The American Medical Association (AMA) has accepted this approach. The AMA's Council of Ethical and Judicial Affairs acknowledges that it is difficult to have a general definition of "medically futile treatments" at the end of life.[2] They recommend what they call a "fair process approach" where there is an open discussion of the medical situation with the patient and/or family participating in the deliberations. They recommend that community standards of medical care be used. The discussion should be about that patient at that time.

A related issue that arises is whether doctors should be authorized to override the patient's wishes to start or continue futile treatments. This is a big question and difficult to answer. As stated above, such decisions should be arrived at by agreement and consensus if at all possible. But in those rare situations when, even after considerable explanation, a patient continues to ask for a treatment that doctors continue to believe is futile, more people can be brought into the conversation. Other medical professionals, clergy and ethicists can meet with the doctors and the patient (or her representatives) to help facilitate mutual understanding of their points of view. The doctors can explain why they consider the treatment to be futile. The patient can explain why, despite the doctors' recommendation, she nonetheless wants that treatment. Such a mediated discussion often leads to better communication between the two groups and resolves the dispute.

All hospitals have ethics committees that help promote such conversations to foster better understanding. If after these discussions the doctor still feels that the treatment should not be given and the patient still wants the treatment, as a last resort, the problem can be referred to a different kind of committee. This could be a committee that includes medical experts not involved in the care of the patient, along with religious and legal professionals and lay people from outside the institution where the patient is being treated. After hearing all sides of the dispute and after due deliberation, this committee would have the authority to make a ruling about whether the treatment should or should not be given or continued.

Such committees with the authority to make a ruling against the medically unrealistic demands of the patient or family have been considered by some institutions but for a variety of reasons are in place only in very few. I give below a possible framework for such a committee, tentatively called the Institutional Care Review Board (ICRB).

If, in the thoughtful, well-grounded judgment of the Institutional Care Review Board, it is determined that life-sustaining treatments would be futile for a given patient, an experienced physician, with concurrence of appropriate colleagues, may withhold such treatments and institute appropriate comfort measures.

The medical team must make all reasonable efforts to convince the patient or his or her surrogate to agree to and understand the reason for such a decision.

Life-sustaining medical treatments include cardio-pulmonary resuscitation, mechanical ventilation, artificial nutrition and hydration, use of blood products, renal dialysis, use of vasopressors, and antibiotics or any other treatment that prolongs the process of dying.

A life-sustaining medical treatment should be considered futile if it cannot be reasonably expected to restore or maintain vital organ function or achieve the expressed goals of the patient when he or she was capable of making decisions.

The attending physician must inform the administration orally and in writing when this policy is invoked and the help of the ICRB is needed.

When a physician feels the need for such support, the physician (attending staff, faculty) would (a) inform the medical staff of his or her assessment of the futility of the treatment and of the support from other staff and (b) document the multiple attempts at communication and explanation of the futility of treatment under discussion for that patient at that time.

In order to implement the policy, the physician needs to:

1. Inform the patient that the Institutional Care Review Board (ICRB) is being called to help resolve the problem. Only the attending physician can initiate the process.
2. Give a copy of this statement to the patient.
3. Ask that a meeting of the ICRB be scheduled allowing sufficient time for the patient and medical team to be able to prepare for and participate in the meeting.

Procedure of the ICRB:

1. The attending physician, the consulting physician and representatives of the patient (and/or the patient) should be given a chance to state their case.
2. The ICRB, after hearing the issues and reasons for or against the treatment, will then deliberate the issues and render its opinion. The three likely decisions are:
   a. The ICRB determines that the treatment should not be continued or initiated. The physician can withhold active treatments. Comfort measures and all other support will be continued.
   b. If the patient does not agree, transfer to another institution, if feasible, can be facilitated. If transfer is not possible, the ICRB's ruling can be implemented after a defined time.
   c. If the ICRB determines that the treatments should be instituted or continued, then the treatment plan will be followed by the same or another physician.

3. *Composition of the Committee*
   a. *Senior physician administrator (e.g., chair of clinical department).*
   b. *Member of the clergy/chaplain appropriate to the patient's belief.*
   c. *Member of the legal profession who is not an employee of the medical facility. A retired judge could be a suitable legal professional.*
   d. *Two members of the ethics committee with a report from the ethics consultation.*
   e. *Another physician with knowledge in the field of the patient's major problem (ad hoc).*
4. *Decision-making*
   a. *The decision of the ICRB will be binding. A two-thirds majority would be required for withholding or withdrawing the treatment.*
   b. *In some cases, the ICRB may refer the case for judicial review.*

A decision made after these steps of consultation, discussion and communication is not casual. It is thought out, and all parties have been given a chance to express their opinions.

Such committees and the approach outlined above are not actually in use, but they are worth considering. This would be an open process. Input from all parties would be given due consideration, and an impartial, informed body would make the decisions. Even without a definition of futile treatment, a decision can be made, after due deliberation, for a given patient taking into account all opinions, hopes and realities. This is consistent with the recommendations of the Institute of Medicine report titled "Dying in America" and issued in September 2014.[3]

Ideally, such a committee would not be needed, and all parties could agree on the course of action after due discussion.

When after due deliberation, discussion and communication, the medical team states that further treatments will not help the patient or the family, it is in everybody's interest to accept that statement and change their goals to comfort and care. It is reasonable to believe doctors when they say that there is nothing more they can do to make a patient recover from an illness and that no further treatments will make the patient better. This does not mean that you as the patient or family member should just accept the doctor's statement without further discussion. The same types of questions that one should ask when a new treatment is offered are appropriate and important when the disease has not responded to treatment and comfort measures are offered rather than active treatment to control the disease.

Questions to ask include: How do you know that the current treatment is not working? Why do you say no further treatments will work? What treatments have you tried? Have you consulted other doctors—at your hospital or experts at another specialized center?

Ask for clarification and be satisfied with the explanations given to you. But once you are fully informed and have thought the situation through, it is best to accept that if the doctor says, "No treatment is available," this is the case. At this point, it is essential that you separate your hopes and wishes from the reality. As stated earlier, hope is very important, but at some point reality has to be accepted. You can shift the focus of your hope from hope for a cure or remission to hope for comfort, peace and high-quality time with loved ones at the end of life.

Accepting that the treatment has not worked is *not a defeat*. Medical science and technology have made major progress, but there are limits to what can be done to reverse the processes that have caused organs to fail. As the disease progresses, one or more organs will not function properly. If the organs are defective to begin with, another insult to the body causes further damage to the previously damaged organ and often to other organs. Once that process begins, it sets up a cycle of events that quickly gets out of control. Multi-organ failure can occasionally be reversed but only if the injury is mild and there is a known and treatable trigger that started the process. Doctors and nurses are trained to reverse some of these acute crises. However, usually very little can be done. There are many ways to keep the patient comfortable and able to interact with his family. Goodbyes can be said, and the patient can die peacefully. Death may come a little sooner than it would have with aggressive treatment, but the person will have loved ones nearby and will avoid suffering from the problems caused by the treatments themselves.

Imagine that you have advanced metastatic cancer. Several vital organs are involved, so surgery is not an option. Your doctors have tried radiation and various chemotherapy agents, but the tumors continue to grow. Next, imagine that you accept another round of chemo with a just-released drug, although this treatment will require that you be hospitalized and will leave you weak and perhaps nauseated. Even if it extends your life by a month or so, you will be likely to feel sick and weak. Now, imagine that, after being informed of the new treatment and its likely side effects, you decide to go home instead. With the help of hospice, you will be largely free of pain and other symptoms. You may have fewer days remaining than you would have had with the treatment, but you spend them in familiar surroundings, with people you love. You feel well enough to enjoy sitting in your garden, to share a laugh with old friends, to go through family photo albums with your grandchildren. If you are religious, your own pastor or rabbi comes by to help you reflect on the meaning of your life and to make peace with your God. Which end would you prefer?

Consider the issues that arise in advanced cancer. As long as the cancer can be controlled by the treatment being given—that is, as long as the tumors do not grow and the cells do not spread to other organs—it is worthwhile to keep trying. In some patients, the time does come when the cancer treatments do not control the disease, but the patient suffers the side effects from them nonetheless. At that time, the cancer has invaded multiple organs, and the organs are not able to function properly. The cancer did not respond to treatment because the cancer cells had become resistant to the drugs. In that circumstance, the most kind and appropriate thing to do is to stop trying to treat the cancer and to pay attention to the patient's comfort. This again is not a "defeat." The nature of cancer is such that in some people it eventually will grow despite their physicians' efforts. Keeping patients comfortable until they die is the best thing the doctors can do for them. It is important to make sure that every reasonable option has been considered and the best effort has been made to treat the cancer, but once this has been done, the goal should shift to comfort and to "quality time." Death will come, but it is doubly sad when futile treatments make it unnecessarily painful for the patient and the family.

Why is it reasonable to accept the doctor's recommendations when he says that no further treatment will work and the patient should be kept comfortable until she dies? In our system of medicine, doctors have been trained to conduct the maximum possible treatments. They are familiar with the latest advances in medicine, and their approach in general is to try every treatment that has any chance of working. For the variety of reasons explained in chapters 8 through 10, doctors do not like to give up. Remember, there are some sociologists who contend that physicians, by their personalities and training, are predisposed to do too much. For this reason, with a patient who is not responding to treatments, rarely do doctors stop treatments if there is any chance of success, small as it may be. Therefore, if the doctor recommends stopping active treatments and providing the patient with comfort care before he dies, it is best to accept this advice.

Another point to note is that the doctors and hospitals make money when they conduct active treatments. They make less money when they give comfort care.

As discussed earlier, there are some groups of people who, for their own reasons, believe that doctors withhold treatments that are available and are effective. Representatives of these groups insist that patients should not give up. They have fixed ideas, and they refuse to see the medical reality. Some of these people are advocates for disabled people. They insist, despite evidence to the contrary, that treatments are withheld from disabled people *because* they are disabled.[4] The reality is that disabled people do, at times, have illnesses for which there is no treatment. For example, a person with multiple sclerosis could develop an aggressive cancer. Doctors withhold treatment from those people because they have no chance of responding to available treatments, not because they happen to be disabled. Attorney Kathryn Tucker, executive director of the Disability Rights Legal Center, is trying to correct certain misconceptions in this area.[5]

Another group are people who have their own peculiar interpretation of their religious texts regarding the sanctity of life. Based on their reading, they believe that patients should not give up medical treatments even if all the evidence clearly shows that no medical treatment would be effective. They ignore medical reality and persuade patients to ask for futile treatments that cause pain and discomfort.

Many medical ethicists and mainstream religious leaders have tried to understand why these people are opposed to comfort before death. Dialogues have been arranged to allow them to explain why they believe doctors withhold treatments. I have read about these people, have had conversations with them and have tried to reason with them. What I have found is a rigid stance, but no rational explanation. They just believe that patients should not give up and that doctors should be forced to give treatments as long as the patient wants them. As a consequence, some states have passed laws that force doctors to treat dying patients actively, despite sound medical reasoning and assessment that the treatment will not work. This is unfortunate. As explained in chapter 3, it is our responsibility as families and health-care providers to prevent these pernicious ideas from becoming a barrier to a comfortable death.

Consequences of Demanding Unrealistic Treatments

Throughout this book, I have used words that have subjective interpretations. They are looked upon differently by each of us. No one can feel what someone else feels about them. The meaning of these words has been discussed and debated by linguists and ethicists for a long time with no definitive outcome or consensus. However, even such subjective words need some elaboration and, more importantly, thought, as we look at the issue of medical futility.

These words are "benefit," "effective" and "reasonable."

In the context of medically futile treatments, these terms need to be accepted as ambiguous. When facing a difficult scenario, they need to be understood as a guide to decisions to be made with due consideration of the patient's total situation. If you feel that being alive for a few more days on life support is a benefit, this is your choice. But it is the responsibility of the doctors to make sure that they explain the full implications of your decision—the pain, the cost and the ultimate futility of the treatment.

If the doctor says that the treatment may be effective, you must ask what the real meaning of "effective" is. Does it mean shrinking a tumor or just stopping its growth for a while? Does it mean control of the disease or just prolonging your life a little longer? Does it mean you will feel better, or will the side effects of the treatment make you suffer?

"Reasonable" is a word that cannot be quantified. We all have our perceptions of "reasonable"; it could be 5 percent or 50 percent. No one can give a number. If you are desperate, 5 percent may be meaningful. At other times 50 percent may not be good enough. Again, when looking at a serious illness, one has to consider what it means when there is a "reasonable" chance of the treatment working. The full implications of the actions need to be taken into account in the process of making a decision.

We have to be satisfied with the lack of clarity of these three words. Most often, we have to work with our "gut feeling." But we can make sure that we have as much information as we can collect, then think about it and work with it. Having some clarity of our goals and values is of great help.

Even in the face of failure of previous treatments and clear evidence that there is no treatment that would help, some people do not accept their situation. Rather than pursuing a path focused on comfort, they demand treatments for the disease. There are many reasons for this. In some cases, it is based on a single issue, but in others multiple forces come into play.

It is worthwhile and important to look into the reasons for the reluctance to change the goal toward comfort in the face of failure of previous treatments. Both doctors and patients (as well as family) are reluctant to accept failure or what they perceive as failure. They feel that accepting failure of treatment is a defeat, so they choose to undertake further active treatments. That is a part of our American culture. However, it is in everyone's interest to look at the situation carefully and consider changing the goal from treatment of the disease to an emphasis on the comfort of the patient and a good death. This may help to reduce painful consequences of active treatments directed at the disease. Not accepting the medical reality is unfortunate and causes distress and harm to all concerned. Accepting reality is not accepting defeat. It is no one's fault. The disease in that patient, the failed organs of the patient, is the cause of the impending death. Understanding that and providing comfort is the realistic, humane way to deal with the situation of progressive disease not responding to active treatments.

The many reasons why doctors over-treat were described earlier. An analysis of why patients and families may *ask* for futile treatments is in order here.

If patients have unrealistic expectations and their doctors want to do their best, the hope and desire of each leads to avoidance of medical reality. In some ways, these mind-sets create a "perfect storm." One's thought and action combine with the other's, and everyone suffers. When the false hopes and desires of each party support each other, the result is that unhelpful treatments are undertaken just because they are available. Also at work may be the attempts, as mentioned earlier, by some religious extremists who push for more treatments because of their interpretation of the sanctity of life.

Poor communication is one common reason why futile treatments are requested. The doctors do not like to give bad news and try to talk around it. Patients and family members may be ready to hear the bad news and accept the reality, but they generally wait for the doctors to initiate this type of conversation. They may feel that talking about a bad outcome may bring it on. So each waits for the other to instigate the discussion.

I believe it is the responsibility of the medical providers—doctors, nurses, social workers and religious personnel—to broach the subject. The conversation should develop slowly, starting with the doctor asking simple questions like: How do you think the situation is developing? What do you think is likely to happen? This opens the way to further questions and exploration of related issues. The patient may ask the doctor to explain what is happening. That provides an opening into one of the most difficult conversations imaginable. At that time, doctors have to be exceptionally honest and truthful. But once the barrier is broken, talking becomes less difficult and the overall medical reality and details follow more easily. Doctors are human, and like almost all humans, they fear death, as chapter 10 noted. This fear of death is real and if not looked at with a realistic perspective can harm both patients and doctors. If both sides yield to this fear, it is likely that the patient will suffer. For the sake of the patient, to prevent unnecessary pain and suffering, this instinctive fear has to be accepted, analyzed and overcome. Patients are more likely to accept bad news if it is presented clearly and sympathetically.

Addressing religious issues is also often avoided, leading patients and their families to ask for futile treatments under the (frequently mistaken) impression that their faith requires them to "do everything" right up to the point of death. Regardless of the patient's beliefs and the doctor's beliefs, both have to be respected and discussed. Openly talking about religious beliefs allows both parties to understand each other better and mutual respect and trust to develop.

Patients frequently refuse to accept the reality of the medical situation because they read about breakthroughs in medicine, they hear about someone who lived when they were expected to die, and they believe in miracles.

Doctors for their part, even with evidence to the contrary, may analyze that evidence with a bias or choose to ignore the facts—because they want to be optimistic. When both parties ignore the evidence, one influencing the other, patients are subjected to treatments that are not in their best interest.

It is common human behavior to think of the exceptions. Similarly, we often rely on our last experience. It is said that generals fight their last war because they are unable to see what is happening at the present time. Patients hear of someone who did well; doctors remember the unusual patient who did better than they expected. Based on these exceptions and anecdotes, they both decide to try more treatments.

Demand for unnecessary treatment is a complex issue, but we will try to examine some of the most common inducements.

a. Hype
b. Hearsay
c. Lack of trust in the medical system
d. Failure to accept medical reality
e. Conviction that "doing is good"
f. Equating acceptance with failure
g. Poor communication by doctors
h. Assumption that someone else pays
i. Suspicion that doctors withhold treatments to save money
j. Surviving spouse
k. Secondary gain
l. Religious organizations
m. Hoping for a miracle
n. Nephew from Chicago

HYPE

We see it in magazines, in newspapers and on television on a regular basis—reports on "cures" and "breakthroughs" for some disease or other and talk about "miracle" drugs and new techniques for diagnosis. The headlines attract attention. The text is somewhat accurate, but still it overplays the real meaning of the medical advance. Most often, the so-called breakthrough is a marginal improvement. The "cure" is actually a small prolongation of life for patients suffering from a particular disease.

There is no question that medical science has made a lot of progress, but it is important to put that progress in perspective. We often hear about the increased life expectancy of Americans, and it is true. What we tend to forget is that the biggest change took place with the implementation of better hygiene and clean water for the majority of people in this country, as I explained earlier in this book. Life expectancy in the early part of the twentieth century on average was low—just 33 years for a person born in 1900—because large numbers of infants and children died of diarrhea, malnutrition and infections. The biggest improvement took place in the 1920s and 1930s due to better living conditions. Subsequently, in the 1940s and 1950s, thanks to antibiotics, control of infections from simple wounds and routine surgery and of diseases like typhoid and tuberculosis made a big impact, as did better care of pregnant women and newborns.

Since the 1960s, improvement has progressed on a much smaller scale. Furthermore, many of the advances have led to changing acute illnesses, such as diabetes, into chronic diseases. Thus, many people are living, but they are not healthy—as people cured of infections were when we first learned how to control bacteria. Keep these facts in mind when you hear of "breakthroughs" in medicine.

The headlines and the overblown stories of medical advances might give you hope, but it could be false hope. The disease described may not be the one you have. For example, there are many kinds of kidney diseases. There may have been some advances in the understanding of one of them, but it may not be yours. Discuss the newspaper article or television report with your doctor and get clarification. If you don't, you may cling to a false hope. Worse, you may trust the article more than your doctor and feel resentful that you are not getting a treatment that you read about. Along with the media, there is also a lot of information on the Internet. You may not be able to separate the nonsense and misinformation from the reasonable. A frank discussion with your doctor will protect you from such hype.

As an aside here, let me address the misleading phrase "a cure for cancer," bandied about by otherwise well-informed members of the public, especially keynote speakers at graduations, who say, for example, "You may not find a cure for cancer, but you can still lead a productive life." Cancer is many different diseases. Although they have certain features in common, such as abnormal cells whose growth often gets out of control (this is what we mean by "malignant"), it is unrealistic for anyone to think that medical science will ever discover a single "cure." Research on cancer involves the painstaking process of addressing the mechanisms that lead to changes in particular types of cancer cells—lung, breast, prostate, etc.—and developing ways to halt their growth or spread. Some researchers study genetic or lifestyle factors that may lead to increased risk of certain kinds of cancer. Some strive to develop treatments that have fewer side effects than those currently available. But no one working in oncology, as a researcher or as a health-care provider, believes that somewhere out there is a one-size-fits-all cure waiting to be found.

In addition to the media themselves, doctors and medical institutions, including medical schools, also put out a lot of hype. In order to be competitive in medicine's business environment, they advertise and promote themselves. Sometimes they exaggerate their achievements even to the point of falsehood. Their goal is to increase their revenue by getting patients to seek treatment at that facility. Since these claims come from established institutions, many patients go to them because they offer hope. The hope and benefit may be real; some patients may be able to get treatments not available elsewhere. They may get better treatment. For some patients, that world-famous medical center might be the best option. It is difficult to separate hype, which is general, from reality, which depends on individual circumstances, goals and values.

From your point of view as a patient, the same approach should be applied as in any patient-doctor interaction. Ask questions. Find out what benefits *you* will get from the special expertise at that facility. Be satisfied that you will benefit. Do not be swayed just by the reputation of the institution. Decide what will help you. For example, if you have a fairly common cancer that was found early, the treatment offered by the cancer center near you might be exactly the same as that provided at one that is world famous. If that is the case, will traveling hundreds of miles, disrupting your family and staying in a hotel provide you with any true benefit?

A March 4, 2013, article in *Time* magazine discussed well-known specialized centers.[1] These institutions publicize, even advertise, the great advances they have made. It is true that they have done a great job; they are responsible for a lot of the progress that has been achieved, and the publicity helps them encourage large contributions from wealthy individuals who want to play a part in defeating disease. But as a patient you need more than general acclaim. What you need to look at is whether you personally will be helped by getting your treatment there. Is it worthwhile to bankrupt your family for a marginal benefit? These centers are expensive, and the treatment may not be covered by your insurance. The same article said that the unethical practices of some institutions demonstrate that their focus is on the money they earn and not necessarily on the benefit to the patient. It is good to get information, but your decision must be based on the reality of your particular situation.

Advocacy groups are another source of hype and exaggeration. There are advocacy groups for many diseases. Kidney, heart, Alzheimer's disease, epilepsy and different types of cancer all have advocacy groups. Perhaps the Susan G. Komen Foundation for breast cancer is the best known. These groups provide a service and help many patients. They provide information to the public and often promote preventive care. At times, they also give financial support to patients in need.

Unfortunately, some organizations that sound noble have been co-opted by commercial entities and businesses that use them for financial gain. As an example, all medical organizations in this country that study the different methods of preventing diseases and diagnosing them early have made clear statements that prostate-specific antigen (PSA) tests should not be conducted in healthy, asymptomatic men for screening purposes. Extensive studies over several years have found that the PSA test causes more harm than good, because false elevation of the antigen is common among many men, not just those with prostate cancer, and finding this elevation leads to additional unnecessary tests and treatments. Despite this clear and universal recommendation, I learned that a group of urologists working with a prostate cancer support group sent out flyers with gas bills in various neighborhoods encouraging men to get this test. Since many men are not aware of the problems that the PSA test can cause, they may get the test and end up with the problems described above. This is an example of a damaging combination of hype and the quest for personal gain.

The Susan G. Komen Foundation raised $472 million in 2011. They sponsor races, walks and a variety of fundraisers. They have virtually monopolized a particular shade of pink. When I was visiting Paris, I saw the iconic Eiffel Tower bathed in Komen-pink light. The foundation has increased awareness about breast cancer, but its basic premise that mammograms save lives has been questioned by major task forces for prevention of disease. The main beneficiaries of routine mammograms as a screening tool are the doctors who perform them. Furthermore, most of the money raised by this foundation is spent on publicity and overhead. Only 16 percent of what they raise goes for research. This was described in detail in an article in the April 25, 2013, *New York Times*.[2]

Publicizing the importance of a good diet, exercise and not smoking has done a lot to reduce the burden and complications of many diseases. Paying attention to changes in the body (such as the development of a lump in the breast) helps patients by allowing early diagnosis and early treatment of many diseases. But raising hopes by false promises does not help patients or the general public. The merging of commercial entities and advocacy groups can cause many problems. They suggest, even push, the idea that there is a medical treatment for every disease and every patient. This is far from the truth. Many diseases, many patients, cannot be cured. But the hype, often for selfish reasons, gives patients and the public false hope that leads to many problems and disappointments. Try to separate hype from reality. Have hope but not false hope.

HEARSAY

People often talk about their illnesses. They talk to family members, friends, neighbors and even people they do not know too well, such as their seatmate on a plane. These conversations bring out personal stories and experiences. If someone is sick or has a sick relative, many people come to share their own information, especially when it is reassuring. They make statements like "I had a friend who was given six months to live, but she is doing well a year later" or "One doctor said there was nothing that could be done, but the specialists in Los Angeles cured him."

Understandably, such anecdotal accounts have a major impact on those who are sick or have a loved one who is. There can be fallacies in these statements. The six months was probably an average. (Only in movies and soap operas do doctors nowadays say, "You have such-and-such amount of time.") A year may be within the normal range of survival of patients with that stage of that particular disease. Prediction of life expectancy is difficult. The patient described also may have had a doctor who was incompetent. For example, he may have mistaken a slow-growing cancer for a fast-growing one. Most importantly, without more details it is not possible to determine if the illness recounted by the friend was the same or even similar to the one that you have.

Again, to avoid false hope, the best solution is to discuss details with your doctor. The people who share their stories with you do it with good intentions—they think they are offering you hope. But medicine and diseases are complex, so the example they give you may or may not be relevant for you. Thank your friends who give you such information, but think about the problem for yourself and make your own decisions based on your understanding of what applies to you.

LACK OF TRUST IN THE MEDICAL SYSTEM

Trust is difficult to develop and easy to lose. This is true in interpersonal relationships, between citizens and politicians, and in life in general. In the medical arena, the same applies. Suppose at a certain time in your interaction with your doctor, you had a misunderstanding. Even if the misunderstanding was resolved, you may continue to have some doubts about your doctor. You may choose to stay with that doctor because the treatment is going well and you are feeling better. Then suppose that, as time goes on, the treatment becomes ineffective and your symptoms and disease return, and the doctor tells you that no further treatment is available. You may have trouble accepting that. This feeling may be exaggerated because of the misunderstanding you had earlier. You should talk to your doctor frankly and say why you do not believe her. Bring your misgivings into the open. Further discussions could clarify the situation, and you could proceed with new plans for management of your condition. If you still have doubts, you can ask to have another doctor take over your care. Work with a doctor you feel comfortable with and one you trust. This is your choice.

Mistrust may occur between a community and a particular medical facility. Some problems can be rectified by communication at an individual level and by clear, honest statements by the institution addressing the reason for the lack of trust. It is possible that there was a report in the newspaper about the hospital where you are being treated. The report described how they had been negligent in the care of a certain patient. This could give you doubts about the hospital as a whole. Rather than rejecting the hospital totally, get more information. Talk to your doctor or ask to talk to someone in the administration of the hospital. If the reported incident was isolated and has been rectified, you will probably be reassured. If you have concerns, ask questions and get clarifications; do not make blanket judgments.

Sometimes whole communities—based on their race, ethnicity, socio-economic status, gender or sexual orientation—develop mistrust not just of individual doctors or institutions but toward medical systems as a whole. One unfortunate reality is that some ethnic or racial groups mistrust the medical profession because of historical realities. In the early years of the opening of the West, many atrocities, including unethical medical practices, occurred. Even into the middle of the twentieth century, Native Americans were discriminated against in medical institutions, and their traditional practices were ignored or criticized. The resulting mistrust has persisted despite the fact that such big-oted approaches are now rare. Many Native Americans still mistrust "Western doctors," even though there are increasing numbers of Native Americans in the medical profession and non-Native physicians are trained to support tra-ditional practices as supplements to Western medicine, provided these prac-tices do not interfere with medical treatments. (For example, a soothing chant might be encouraged, while a tea made from an herb that interacts badly with a prescribed medication would not.) This mistrust commonly manifests itself as a perception that treatments are withheld from Native Americans because of their ethnicity—that a white person would get more or better treatments. Further, some Native Americans believe that doctors consider members of their community to be less valuable.

African Americans have suffered a long history of discrimination in our society. Until the mid-1960s, in parts of the country, African Americans had to seek their care at segregated hospitals that had inferior facilities and services. To make matters worse, some groups of unethical physicians misled many patients into research studies without their permission or even adequate infor-mation. The worst of these was the Tuskegee experiment, in which a number of black males with syphilis were deliberately not treated, although effective treatment for the disease was available. This was purportedly so that research-ers could study the "natural progression" of syphilis. Change has occurred, and many African American leaders, health-care professionals and columnists are urging their community to understand that medical discrimination based on race is rare now.

Other minority groups have had similar experiences, but it is not clear if the discrimination was due to ethnicity or to socioeconomic factors. According to an Institute of Medicine report, many medical institutions will not treat patients on Medicaid, and that adds to the feelings of discrimination.[3]

An article in the *Journal of the American Medical Association* discusses the problem of health care disparity in the United States.[4] It points out that even though segregation was outlawed in the 1960s by the passage of civil rights laws, an implicit racial bias persists in our society, as the deaths of Michael Brown at the hands of police officers in Ferguson, Missouri, and Trayvon Martin by a neighborhood watch volunteer in Miami Gardens, Florida, illustrate.

African Americans and other minorities have less access to health care, and they have worse outcomes for common medical problems like diabetes, high blood pressure and diseases related to smoking. The article explains that these differences are related to other problems in society like poverty, inferior education and poor housing. It goes on to recommend, "Medical schools, health care organizations, and credentialing bodies should pay greater attention to disparities in health and health care as a national priority. These organizations should redouble their efforts to increase awareness of disparities, enhance diversity in the health professions, and work toward eliminating discrimination and its adverse effects on health and health care. Considerable evidence is available to guide in the implementation of interventions to reduce racial/ethnic differences in health and health care."

An effort is being made by social scientists and government to correct these problems. At my medical school, there is an associate dean for disparity. He is an African American charged with implementing these needed changes.

Another reason for disparity in health care is sexual orientation. Lesbians, gays, and bisexual and transgender individuals have been discriminated against, but this is happening less.

There is a paradox in the way the poor and the marginalized segments of society are affected by the health-care system in general and at the end of life. Robert Truog, who teaches medical ethics at Harvard, points out that people in these groups get poor health-care services: "Futility cases most commonly involve patients and families from more marginalized and disadvantaged segments of society. These are families who have lived on the outskirts of our health-care system and who have frequently been denied or perceive they have been denied care that is beneficial."[5]

Unfortunately, this situation is reversed at the end of life. Preethy Nayar of the University of Nebraska School of Public Health found that patients who identified as racial minorities had more ICU days, emergency room visits and inpatient days than non-Hispanic whites—an unfortunate aspect of our system.[6]

The impact of these practices by some, especially in the past, is difficult to quantify. But sociologists have noted that patients in these communities are more likely to demand treatments that doctors tell them will not work.[7] These patients often feel that treatments are withheld from them because of their socioeconomic situation or their race or ethnicity. It is harder to convince them that the treatment is being withheld because of medical reasons. Similar suspicion is seen among those who are older or have some form of disability. Again, they do not accept that at a certain point medical treatments do not work or may be inappropriate for them. In fact, age and disability may themselves reduce the chances of the treatment being effective. A treatment should be withheld only if it is not going to work, but not just on the basis of age or disability.

This mistrust is manifested most commonly at the end of life when a patient with multiple, advanced medical problems is advised not to have CPR. Because of suspicion of discrimination, seriously ill low-income or minority patients insist on CPR in the event that their hearts stop. They do not accept that the only thing that CPR would do is to increase pain for the patient and family. The reality of CPR is misunderstood by many people who feel that treatments, including CPR, are being withheld in order to save money. Such suspicion is unfortunate but understandable. Detailed discussion and explanation is the only way to avoid further hardship. If doctors are sensitive to the patient's and family's perception, they can and should talk about it openly and then emphasize the medical reality of a futile treatment. If the patient continues to suspect that she is being discriminated against for non-medical reasons, the doctors should address that concern honestly and explain that the treatment, in this case CPR, is not advisable because it most likely will not work, regardless of the patient's race or socioeconomic situation. Socioeconomic factors should not determine the doctor's decision, and rarely do. For some families, bringing in a doctor of the same ethnicity as the patient helps.

If you feel a lack of trust in your medical team, express yourself. Do not assume that you are being denied treatments because of your socioeconomic situation or your background. Have the doctors give you all the information you need to accept the futility of the treatment.

FAILURE TO ACCEPT MEDICAL REALITY

Optimism and hope are major coping mechanisms. These emotions, combined with overly positive statements one hears in every walk of life, take us away from reality and acceptance. We want a fix for anything that is not working well. We fail to appreciate the cost of the fix—in pain, side effects and the psychological price of trying treatments that will not help.

Refusal to give up is a part of the American mind-set. Studying hard to understand a difficult problem in school, solving challenging dilemmas at work, striving extra hard to save our job or the company we run are good. These situations offer a reasonable chance of success. The cost of the hard work, in itself, is not devastating.

It is difficult to change our attitude when dealing with a life-threatening illness. The stakes are very high. Some patients will die. This is obviously not an easy situation for the patient or the family and friends. But does denial of the reality help? Does persisting in our struggle do any good? Death is inevitable. The issue is accepting that basic fact at the time when it faces you. Whatever your religious beliefs, your economic status or your hope, the medical reality does not change. How is the medical reality determined? By factual information, by the condition of the patient's vital organs and the status of the disease. Understanding each of these components has to be the first step. You do not have to know science or medicine to understand these. Talking to your doctor to get clear answers is what is key. Like you, doctors do not want to give up. They want to do everything possible within reasonable limits. They know what to do and what not to do. Trust, as stated above, is difficult to develop. But when you have trusted your doctors with your or your loved one's treatment, should you not trust them with the determination of the limits of medical treatments? Doctors have nothing to gain by wrongly or prematurely stopping or withholding treatments.

Accepting failure is difficult, but sometimes it has to be done. Is it really a failure? Whatever the cause of the illness, whatever the nature of the disease, one has to keep in mind that we all have to die. Acceptance of reality is a great service to the patient. Acceptance of death, after due deliberation, is the biggest gift we can give to ourselves and our loved ones. Acceptance and trust are both difficult but do go hand in hand when dealing with life-threatening situations and death. What gets in the way of acceptance is false hope or wishful thinking. If based on a false premise, hope is false hope. Wishful thinking helps one deal with the initial impact of bad news, but it does not change the course of events.

As hard as it may be, for the sake of all concerned, examine why you are not accepting reality.

Your medical providers, as I stated earlier, have many reasons to urge treatments. Their hope, their way of thinking and the health-care system all push them to do more and more. So when they say there are no further treatments for the disease, it will be after all options have been looked at and tried. This is the time to consider other ways of dealing with the situation, the time when your goal needs to change. The new goal should be for comfort during the precious time remaining to you and the opportunity to prepare for a comfortable death.

The reasons for holding onto false hope are many. They are personal. Each individual, whether patient or family member, has his or her own reasons. If you as the patient persist in wanting to try yet another treatment, you need to look inward. Why do I not believe the doctors when they say that no treatment is available? You need to look at the full picture. Yes, talk to the doctor again, ask questions, but ultimately only you can accept the medical reality.

Accepting the reality of progressive disease and vital organs that are not functioning allows the patient to die peacefully.

CONVICTION THAT "DOING IS GOOD"

It is a part of our thinking in all aspects of life: Doing something about a problem is always better than doing nothing. But doing something that is useless and harmful is not a good practice. In fact, in some situations action causes more trouble than inaction. We have the mind-set that to do something when faced with a problem is good, but doing something for the sake of doing is not. Sure, when action needs to be taken, when doing something can be beneficial, it must be done.

We have been brought up to believe that we must always do our best. This is a good general rule. It applies to medicine. If a patient suffers a stroke or an injury, efforts at rehabilitation are needed. The harder we work to strengthen our muscles and to keep our joints mobile, the better the recovery. Undergoing painful surgery to remove an inflamed appendix is doing something good. But doing something when all evidence, all previous experience, shows that it will not work is a misapplication of the rule. Sometimes "doing our best" means doing less. Acceptance of reality at a certain point is helpful and comforting.

EQUATING ACCEPTANCE WITH FAILURE

Acceptance of reality is the best way to achieve peace of mind. Of course, we must make sure that what we are accepting is real. Full analysis of the situation and understanding of the medical facts must come first.

But once it is clear that no medical treatment will control the disease, acceptance of that reality will provide solace and comfort. It will allow you to change your goals, to think of other ways to deal with a sad situation. It will allow you and your family to come closer, and death will be peaceful. Change of goals toward comfort and closure helps everyone.

Changing our goals in this way is not failure; it is coming to terms with a situation over which we have no control. We all have to accept realities that are not pleasant. Divorce, loss of a job and income, and damage to our property in natural disasters are unfortunately common. The consequences are not pleasant, but we accept them and make the choices we need to make. We may have tried to compromise, but once we lose our job, for example, we have to go on from there. Acceptance of reality and working out the best path forward is what helps. Recognizing that the disease cannot be controlled opens the path to comfort for the patient and solace for the family and friends.

As mentioned earlier in the book, there are some who teach and preach the opposite. It is difficult to identify these people, but there are many, and they push their idea in many ways. Through their speech and writing, they make it difficult for the patient and family to get comfort physically and emotionally. Some of these zealots publicize the idea that the reason the treatment failed was that the patient did not try hard enough. They claim that diseases can be controlled by sheer willpower. What this does is to add guilt to the patient's other burdens. The claim is obviously meaningless. Yes, willpower may allow you to deal with the situation more effectively, but it cannot control the disease—certainly not advanced or terminal illness.

Many proselytizers and self-help gurus come under this category. Their claims are based not on religion or spirituality but on unrealistic extrapolation and in many cases are a mechanism for self-promotion. There is a physician who happened to have cancer and was cured—a phenomenon that is not rare for the type of cancer he had. Whether it was the nature of his cancer or the treatment that led to his cure is not clear. However, this doctor, Bernie Segal, claimed that he was cured because of his willpower, courage and what he called positive thinking—a meaningless and baseless claim.[8] He struck a chord with a segment of the population, made many speeches, wrote books, appeared on TV and made a lot of money. In the process, he gave false hope to and hurt many people. One major disservice he did was to blame the victim. He implied that if your cancer was not cured, it was your fault. If it were that simple, this approach would have changed the world.

If you are facing an aggressive serious illness and treatments to control the disease have failed, redefine "positive thinking" in your own terms to apply to the pleasures and successes you have enjoyed in life, to the love and companionship of your family and friends, and to peace and comfort in whatever time you have left.

POOR COMMUNICATION BY DOCTORS

There are many doctors who are great communicators. They give presentations at medical conferences. They speak clearly when they discuss cases with their colleagues. They are also good at explaining the disease as well as the plan and science behind treatments to patients and families. They are confident and serve this function well.

However, when it comes to explaining to patients that no further potentially effective treatments remain for them, these same physicians often find this part of their communication role extremely difficult. Their mind-set, their training, and the competitive environment they work in may all contribute to their discomfort. Whatever the reason, many physicians are unable to give bad news. They are not dishonest, they understand the situation, but they are unable to tell the patient that the treatments that were tried have not worked and that no other good options are available.

A senior colleague of mine, an oncologist like me, has excellent medical skills and a great fund of knowledge, and he is a compassionate person. I have heard him on several occasions describe how a patient had a good response to a particular treatment but the cancer started to grow back again. He was disappointed but acknowledged to his colleagues that further treatment of the cancer would not be effective and comfort care would be the patient's best option. However, when it comes to working with the patient, this otherwise fine physician does not—or cannot—follow through on this assessment and the approach he recommends to others. Instead, he calls on his great fund of knowledge to find some treatment that "may" work or some research study in which the patient could participate. Through this approach, he continues to treat the patient until the patient is too ill even to walk a few steps into the clinic. Many nurses have noted that this oncologist's patients have been given therapy when they were very weak and sick.

When physicians fail to face the reality that the treatments that were tried did not work and that it is time to switch the goal from defeat of the disease to comfort, they deprive you and your family of a chance to deal calmly with the end. If the physician does not communicate the reality to the patient, the patient continues to have hope for cure or substantial remission—false hope. The doctor's evasion of reality gives the patient the idea that she should ask for and try more treatments.

ASSUMPTION THAT SOMEONE ELSE PAYS

In our country pay for medical treatments is based on a fee-for-service system. All doctors, all institutions and all drug companies need to be paid. There are ways to make some adjustments, but ultimately someone has to pay for treatments and procedures.

If you have medical insurance, private or through the government (e.g., Medicare or Medicaid), that will cover many of the costs. But there is often a co-pay or a deductible. The insurance pays for a part, and the patient has to pay the rest. The system is complex. Different interventions are covered or not covered, the co-pay and deductibles vary from plan to plan, but patients in most cases do have a financial responsibility that can add up to a significant amount. For example, your insurance may pay for hip replacement surgery, perhaps with a $2,000 deductible, but only cover half of the time your doctors recommend in a rehabilitation center. Doctors in general do not discuss the cost of the treatment with patients.

If you do not have insurance, you are responsible for the entire payment. Those providing the service may help you set up a payment plan, or they may defer charges, but you are still responsible.

Medical bills are the leading cause of personal bankruptcy in this country.

In July 2015, the American Society of Clinical Oncology (ASCO) published a statement on the cost and "value" of treatments for cancer.[9] This represents a major advance in the approach of the oncology community toward addressing the issue of cost of cancer treatments to individuals and to society as a whole.

The statement points out that because of the recent availability of some new and very expensive drugs, the rise in the cost of cancer chemotherapy is greater than the increase in cost in other fields of medicine. It also reiterates the problems of bankruptcy due to the financial burden of medical treatments and points out that many patients are surprised and unprepared for high out-of-pocket expenses.

ASCO is encouraging the oncology community at large to assess the "value" of cancer therapy for their patients. This includes finding a balance between clinical benefit (efficacy), toxicity (safety) and cost (efficiency). This is a complex balancing act, and the society is seeking feedback to formulate a usable system. It is a good beginning. ASCO is also encouraging oncologists to include talking to patients about the cost of treatments along with discussing needs, goals and preferences that could affect their decisions.

The Institute of Medicine and the American College of Physicians have started such initiatives, as well.

These discussions within the profession are good beginnings, but the sometimes unmanageable costs borne by patients and their families continue.

If the treatment has a reasonable chance of making you well again, such an economic burden is worthwhile. But to risk financial ruin and to deprive your family of scarce resources in order to take a treatment that has only limited chances of helping for a short time probably is not. You need to think about this before asking for treatments that you "hope" will help.

It would be sad if someone with a decent chance of recovery were denied treatment because he could not pay for it. Fortunately, in most developed countries, this is rare. Effective and reasonable treatments are available to most people. When it comes to treatments that have a small chance of bringing about recovery, or when the patient has an illness that would leave her chronically ill or unable to function, the medical systems in many countries place restrictions on how much is paid and what treatments are used.

This limitation is more common in countries in Europe, where the government pays for a large part of the treatment and thus has a stake in preserving limited resources for those who would benefit the most—for example, a child with a treatable leukemia, rather than an elderly person with lung cancer that has metastasized to the brain.

In these countries, patients sometimes may wait many months for procedures that are not necessary to their survival, although they have a high chance of improving quality of life. For example, a friend of a friend, who lives in New Zealand, had to wait close to a year for a hip replacement. While she waited, she could still get around, albeit with a cane. Once her turn for the surgery came up, however, the government covered the full cost of the surgery and the rehabilitation. People in countries with such restrictions are free to travel abroad for prompter treatment, but they must pay the costs out of pocket.

In the United States, questions about the outcome or suitability of treatment are generally not decided on the basis of cost. The decision is made between the patient and family and the medical provider. The doctors do not want to restrict tests and treatments based on economic considerations, at least not with price as the main parameter. Even though ultimately doctors and hospitals do get paid for the treatments they provide, they try to be careful when it comes to treatments with small chance of benefit. Some do inform the patient about the chance of benefit as well as the financial cost he may have to bear.

The patient or the family does not want to place a monetary value on a life, but the situation is not simple. They need to understand three important aspects of this complex problem. First is how likely that treatment (at that time in that patient) is to be effective and to what degree. At least they need to know generally if the chances are good, in between or poor. Next they need to understand how functional, productive and comfortable the patient would be even if the treatment were to work. Quality of life is an important parameter when making treatment decisions. The factor to be considered third, but not to be ignored, is the cost, both the total cost and an estimate of what the patient and family's share would be after the third party (insurance, etc.) pays for whatever is covered. Add to these the expense of after-care. Will a family member need to quit a job or take an extensive unpaid leave of absence in order to provide assistance with all the tasks of daily living, or will the family need to pool resources to hire home health aides round the clock? Typically, insurance provides nothing, or only a small fraction, of such expenses. No answer is clear-cut or certain; it is qualitative or at best semi-quantitative. However, these issues need to be discussed and given due thought and consideration before treatment decisions are made.

To illustrate the point I will describe two specific scenarios. If an otherwise healthy 22-year-old develops a heart problem that has a good chance (say 70 percent) of being corrected, and the patient is likely to lead a satisfactory life after the surgery, almost everyone would agree that the treatment is justified and worthwhile. Even if the operation cost $50,000 and the family did not have the resources, it would be considered a good decision to go ahead with it and deal with the financial issues later.

Take as another example a 60-year-old with damaged lungs and heart who spent the last year at home in bed on oxygen. This patient now develops a new problem in the liver. Treatment of the liver problem would not fix the problems with the heart or lungs. The treatment for the liver disease may or may not be effective, and it would cost the family $30,000, which they do not have. In this situation, as a physician, I would have an open, detailed discussion with the patient and family and inform them of the reality. I would ask them to consider whether it would be worthwhile to go into debt for the sake of a treatment that would make no real difference to the outcome. The decision would be theirs, but they would need to understand the full situation.

Do not place a price tag on Grandma, but do think about and discuss the issue. In fact, bringing Grandma into the conversation would be helpful. She may decide not to take the treatment because she would rather die knowing that her limited remaining resources will be available to send her grandchildren to college.

SUSPICION THAT DOCTORS WITHHOLD TREATMENTS TO SAVE MONEY

As stated above, ours is a fee-for-service system. Even if doctors and hospitals provide treatments that don't help, they will charge for them, and they will do their best to recover the charges. At a purely financial level, it is in an institution's interest to do as many procedures as they can rationalize. It is the doctors' honesty that keeps them from doing too much just for financial gain. But if you demand a treatment, they may be justified in giving it to you, and they will earn money from it. Most doctors will discourage you from undertaking a procedure or treatment if it is not appropriate. But if you insist, they will go ahead and provide it, and they will be paid for it—either by your insurance company or, if it denies approval, by you. So doctors do not save money by withholding a treatment they consider futile. In fact, they make money by doing the opposite.

There are situations where insurance companies put limits on how long a patient can be in the hospital. If the patient has an incurable illness and has been hospitalized for a long time, the insurer may refuse to pay to extend the stay in an acute care hospital. Depending on the specifics of the disease and the chances of recovery, the patient may benefit from transfer to a rehabilitation facility or nursing home or be eligible for comfort care with the help of hospice. Many physicians send the patient to rehabilitation facilities rather than hospice. By doing so the doctor avoids the difficult conversation about death and the incurability of the illness. Although the physician transfers her responsibility to the rehabilitation center or nursing home, the burden on you or your family is not lessened. The long-term-care facility benefits financially from keeping you there, because your stay there is usually covered by Medicare and Medicaid.

SURVIVING SPOUSE

Many people want their ill spouses to undertake or continue aggressive treatments because they are afraid to live without them. After living with and loving each other for decades, these husbands and wives cannot imagine a life for themselves alone.

From a friend, I heard the story of a devoted husband whose wife had advanced cancer. He was well-off financially and felt he should help his wife to get any treatment available anywhere in the country. The wife did not want to exhaust herself traveling and enduring experimental treatments. She wanted to be at home and spend her limited remaining time with her family and friends. However, she did not want her husband to feel that she was abandoning him by "giving up." The husband, for his part, remembered that his elderly mother had died about a decade earlier in a car crash with his father driving. The husband's father survived without serious injuries but felt tormented by guilt for the remaining five years of his life. The devoted husband thought that if he did not seek every possible treatment for his wife, he would be "causing" her death, almost as clearly as his father had caused his mother's.

The couple first went to the world-famous M.D. Anderson Cancer Center in Houston. After evaluating the wife, the doctors at Anderson said there was no standard treatment available for her. Even after they advised her that the experimental study currently underway had little potential for benefiting her personally, she enrolled in it and then in another study at Sloan Kettering in

New York. After neither of these treatments significantly halted the growth or spread of her cancer, she returned to M.D. Anderson. This time, the doctors explained that she was now too sick to qualify for their experimental protocols.

Upon hearing this news, the husband became so angry at the doctors at M.D. Anderson that he even threatened legal action against them. He then took his wife back to the Sloan Kettering Cancer Center in New York and to the University of California, Los Angeles. Both gave the same answer—there was no treatment for the wife's cancer.

He finally accepted the reality, and his wife died at home. This is an example of a loving, devoted husband who could not face the death of his wife and, in the process, took her around the country seeking treatments that obviously were futile.

For decades, I have had three close friends, each of whom has had a good marriage, loving and caring. All were in good health. About seven years ago one of the men, who was full of life and spirit, was found to have kidney cancer that had spread to other parts of his body. He was a doctor and initially tried the most aggressive treatments available. But the cancer kept progressing. After a while, he and his wife decided that he should go for comfort care, and he died peacefully in his home. His children, grandchildren and friends were all there. His memorial service was a celebration of his vibrant life.

This was the first death among my circle of friends. We were concerned about how the wife would cope with the loss of her husband. She had the support of her children, brothers and extended family. She adjusted to the change. She and all of us continue to remember our friend and his life—his faux pas, his habits and his spirit. Gradually, she developed her own life and met another man, and her life goes on.

The rest of us in our circle remain generally healthy in our sixties and seventies. We talk about our deaths but enjoy our lives. Sure, when one of the group dies, we will miss him or her. The couples have not known any life except with their spouses. No one can predict how the surviving spouse will do. But we all feel that keeping the one who is dying "alive" is not in anyone's interest. We accept death, accept that there will be a major change after the death of one of us. But the surviving spouse will continue to have a life—a different life, but a life. To keep a dying person on life support or on painful ineffective treatments would be selfish. Such a path does not prolong life but just prolongs the dying process.

Unfortunately, many spouses are so afraid of "change" that they ask their partner to undergo treatments that are painful and of no benefit. They even want their husband or wife to undergo painful, isolating treatments in the ICU rather than spending the last few days together. Misguided hope is the main reason for these demands for futile treatments. Love, combined with pressure from, among others, family, news media hype and religious groups reinforces this negative behavior. The surviving spouse needs to be supported, needs love and tenderness, and needs to be counseled regarding the inevitability of death.

Widowhood is difficult, especially if the marriage was happy and caring. Recently, two well-known women writers, Joan Didion and Joyce Carol Oates, were widowed, and each has written eloquently of her adjustment. Both had loving relationships and both were devastated.[10] But both could cope with the change and continued to write. They describe their emotions and their lives after the deaths of their husbands. Although it has not been easy, they continue to be active and productive. Oates wrote, "Of the widow's countless death duties there is really just one that matters: on the anniversary of her husband's death the widow should think: I kept myself alive." Staying alive is not easy because it involves surmounting fears and anxieties for which there is no training. The point is that the healthy spouse must give due importance to the medical facts and reality of the sick one. Decisions regarding starting or continuing treatments must be based on an understanding of the reality after discussion with the medical team.

A very important point that was made earlier is worth repeating. If the doctors suggest comfort measures, rather than a trial of another treatment, it is most likely that, even if successful in the short term, the treatment will not return the spouse to the health he enjoyed before the crisis. If he is so seriously sick that all standard treatments have failed, the chances are that you will not get your spouse back. He will continue to need care and support, and life is not going to be as it was. Think of the consequences for your spouse and for yourself before demanding a futile, ineffective treatment. If the couple are of advanced age, the burden of caring for the spouse can be detrimental to the well-being and health of the surviving spouse. If you are the patient, causing such hurt to your spouse based on unrealistic hope may be selfish.

Correspondingly, some sick people want to continue treatments because they do not want to abandon their spouses. In both cases, the chances are that even if the sick one survives, she is likely to be too chronically unwell to interact in a meaningful way. It is so much more kind to say "I love you," say your goodbyes and accept death.

SECONDARY GAIN

In some circumstances, there is a secondary gain just to keeping a patient alive. A friend of mine was head of a dialysis unit at a Veterans Administration hospital. Over the years, he had patients on long-term dialysis. Some patients had poor quality of life; they had other medical problems, and they were willing to die. However, the patients told my friend that as long as they were alive, their wives would get veterans' benefits. For this reason, they decided to continue with the dialysis.

In this case, a futile treatment was continued just to provide financial help to the family of a patient who was ready to die.

These are special circumstances, and we need to give that due respect, but even here there are limits, and we need to accept them.

RELIGIOUS ORGANIZATIONS

As described in chapter 3, personal faith, belief and religion provide solace, comfort and a sense of closure and acceptance when dealing with a sad and difficult situation. However, some religious organizations sometimes interfere with the families' feelings and values. They rely on their doctrines. The doctrines have rigid rules, often laid down long before the present, when the world was different. For example, many medical therapies that are now common— intravenous feeding, respirators, chemotherapy—had yet to be invented. Since there was no technology for life support, these long-held doctrines do not address anything for the seriously ill beyond prayer, spoon-feeding, comfort care and (for some religions) a prohibition against actively hastening death. But some people cling to rules that are not relevant to our time. For families facing serious illness and death, it is important to base decisions and actions on their personal faith, informed by their acceptance of medical reality, and not to be swayed by outsiders' rules and convictions that may not be applicable to them.

A friend of mine is the pastor of a church. He has strong faith and beliefs. Over the past several months, he and I have talked about death and my efforts to make every death a comfortable, good death. After we had had this conversation a few times, he said, "When I am seriously ill, I want you to help me die comfortably. If it is in God's will, God will work through you to make my death comfortable." He told me that he even would accept Aid in Dying (AiD), described in this book's last chapter, if that were appropriate.

HOPING FOR A MIRACLE

When faced with a catastrophic situation, it is common to seek hope. One of the ways people get hope is by believing that there can be a "divine intervention." The concept of divine intervention is personal and cannot be defined. Regardless, a Harris Poll conducted in 2013 found that 74 percent of Americans believe in divine miracles.[11]

Thus, having belief or hope for a miracle is in a sense normal. The root of such a hope is unclear. It may be based on stories about someone who recovered from a serious illness when they were not predicted to. It may come from situations where the facts were not accurately stated or understood. Also it could be due to "good luck." Separating these is difficult in medical situations. Yet people believe in or hope for miracles. I should add that I am not in a position to comment on the miracles performed by Jesus (such as Lazarus being raised from the dead), and that I have to leave these to theologians. What I can say is that some groups read these miracles metaphorically and others see them as real events. The progress in medical technology and success in treating some patients who were expected not to recover is one factor that may lead people to use the word "miracle." The word is employed rather loosely in day-to-day interactions Have you heard a friend say something like "I left my purse in the restaurant, and when I went back, it was a miracle that it was still there." Yes, some patients recover when not expected to. Also, patients may have an overly pessimistic idea of their prognosis; for example, they may consider any diagnosis of cancer a death sentence. When the treatment is effective, they are surprised and may call it a miracle. I have been credited with performing "miracles" when all I did was to use a standard treatment on a patient who had a treatable disease.

Confusing the above-mentioned scenarios with the situation faced by a patient who has an advanced disease that has not responded to the best available treatments can cause problems. If a patient has multiple organs that are damaged and the condition is getting worse despite treatments, expecting a miracle is not in the interest of the patient or yourself as a family member. Make sure all that can and should be done has been done. If the doctors say nothing more can be done, accept that. Don't expect a miracle, but if it gives you consolation, hope for a miracle. That hope can be comforting.

It is one thing to *hope* for a miracle; however, making your decisions because you *expect* a miracle can only hurt all concerned. By their nature, miracles are very rare exceptions; we should not rely on them or base our actions on them. Those who believe in miracles also believe that miracles are divine actions and are not performed by humans. Those who believe in praying for a miracle to save a person's life should do so if this offers consolation and hope. But to plan your actions or make your decisions based on the hoped-for occurrence of a miracle is not in your or your family's best interest. We have to accept that we all will die.

Interestingly, it has been observed that nonreligious people also get solace when they hope for a miracle.

THE NEPHEW FROM CHICAGO

Sometimes relatives show up when a patient is sick. Often these visitors have little understanding of the situation; nonetheless, they force their personalities onto the family, demanding treatments that they may have vaguely heard of. Such information may have no bearing on the patient's illness, but it could lead to demand for treatments that will not help.

The family members who have been with the sick relative on a day-to-day basis are more likely to accept that death is near. They understand the sick person's suffering. They are willing to let the patient die in peace. Those relatives who did not know or understand what had happened or was happening to the patient are more likely to demand more treatments, in a misguided desire to help. Sometimes they have guilty feelings about not being there when the family member got sick. They may try to compensate for their absence by demanding extra treatments. If they happen to live in one of the metropolitan centers (New York, Chicago, Los Angeles) and the patient is being treated in a smaller city (Des Moines or Albuquerque), they may consider the local medical facility backward and inadequate. As a result they may push the family and doctors into further treatments that only hurt the patient. The family should work together. Everyone should understand the reality of what is going on with the patient—the illness, what treatments have been tried, and what is happening at that time. It is not helpful to let someone who is not familiar with the full story guide your decisions. It may help to have the "nephew" meet with the doctors.

As in many situations surrounding serious illness, clear, informed and compassionate communication will result in the best outcome for everyone involved. Patients and their families and friends want the sick person to live long and have her disease treated and thereby controlled or cured. Doctors want the same for the patient. But there are limitations, and these goals cannot be met in every case. The situation should be discussed among the doctors and the patient and family, goals set, and treatment planned and implemented. Usually the goals are realistic, the plan feasible and the treatment effective.

Of course, this cannot happen every time. Sometimes the goals are not met; the treatment is not effective. Then the goals need to be modified according to the new reality. At this point, the doctor and the patient will be disappointed, but usually all the parties will be able to reassess and readdress the current status of the disease and the patient. Some participants may accept the reality and modify goals based on the new circumstances determined by the disease, the patient's general health status and the availability of effective treatments. They recognize that there are limits to medicine and that the most prudent course is to change the goal of treatment to providing the patient with comfort and palliation without further attempts to control the disease.

There are no defined limits, no rules and no clear criteria as to when one should, can or must change the goal to comfort for the patient and when to continue attempts to control the disease. Each situation is unique, but there are some generalizations that do apply.

Sometimes doctors or patients, for a variety of reasons, may not want to change goals and may want to continue treatments aimed at controlling the disease. Outsiders cannot interfere with that decision. However, continuing treatments just for the sake of continuing can cause problems. If not faced sensitively, openly and honestly, many factors come together and lead to a frame of mind that focuses on active treatments even against poor odds. Comfort for the patient before the virtually inevitable death is forgotten.

Some of the consequences of these treatments are worth looking at. They include the following:

a. Prolongation of the patient's pain and discomfort
b. Separation of the patient from loved ones when they are needed the most
c. Regrets
d. Conflicts within the family

e. Medical bills you may need to pay (co-pays and deductibles)

f. Long-term recovery and stress on caregivers

g. Uncertainty

Prolongation of the Patient's Pain and Discomfort

If you as the patient undertake a treatment for a disease that is advanced or not likely to respond to further treatments, you will suffer not only from the effects of the disease but also from the side effects of the treatment, such as nausea, vomiting, dizziness and the problems due to the administration of the treatment or to performing the tests. Even traveling to and from the clinic can be a burden if you feel sick or exhausted.

Treatments in these circumstances can be painful. Enduring pain for a short time with a good chance of recovery is worthwhile and justified. But pain caused in the pursuit of a false hope is not in your interest. When doctors undertake such treatments, they are obligated to follow the patient closely with monitoring, blood tests and X-rays—all of which can cause significant distress. Sometimes the use of medications to relieve pain has to be restricted if the patient is receiving active treatments. Delay in implementing comfort measures may cause more distress.

By undertaking a treatment just because of hope, you may feel satisfied that you did your best. But once again, for the sake of all concerned, if the treatment is not working, discuss that with your doctors and stop. Focus on your comfort and the well-being of your family.

Treatments based on false hope only prolong the dying process. They do not give additional life to the patient. They make death painful.

Separation of the Patient from Loved Ones When They Are Needed the Most

Just being in the hospital isolates the patient from his family. One family member may be allowed to stay overnight with the patient, but the number of visitors allowed in the room even during the day will be limited, if only by the size of the space.

In the ICU, the isolation and discomfort are magnified. The term "intensive care unit" is in some ways misleading. The personnel may be very caring, but because of the nature of what needs to be done, there is a lot of *treatment*. As mentioned in chapter 8, some suggest the facility should be called the intensive treatment unit (ITU), rather than the ICU.

Treatment in the ICU usually involves many types of tubes and intravenous lines; these will have monitors attached to them to check the status of the patient's oxygen levels, heart function, temperature and blood pressure. Nurses and doctors will be required to be with the patient constantly. The family will be allowed to visit with their seriously ill loved one only for short periods. Young children, including the grandchildren and great-grandchildren who could give the patient a precious sense of continuity, will typically be excluded. Because of the sedation usually needed, visitors will not be able to communicate clearly with the patient. This isolation is required for the ICU team to perform their jobs properly, but it can be distressing to the family.

Even treatments outside the ICU can be isolating. The side effects of the treatment may force the patient to remain confined. If, on the other hand, the goal is shifted to comfort before death, the patient can often be at home, in reassuringly familiar surroundings, with family, friends and even pets around. The family will have a better chance to come close, talk about the patient's life, say goodbyes and share their lives. If needed, they can share emotions that were not shared earlier. This helps to bring closure.

Regrets

As a patient, you may have regrets about your decision if you continue active treatments, especially if you do not improve on them. You may ask yourself "Why am I doing this?" If that time comes, you do have the option of stopping the treatment. Continuing the treatment is up to you. If you feel it has not done what you hoped for, talk to your medical team; they can explain what can be done to change the plan. You will still have the satisfaction that you tried your best and will still have the benefit of spending time with your family before your death, which will now be more likely to be comfortable. If you made the decision to undertake a treatment with a low chance of working, that is okay. If you made that decision after thinking through the issues, after understanding the pros and cons, you will have fewer regrets. We all have made decisions in our lives that in retrospect were not good ones. If you make a medical treatment decision without thinking about it fully, you may have more regrets than if you carefully considered the pros and cons.

At a certain stage, aggressive medical treatment can become sanctioned torture. But as health-care professionals, our mind-set may be such that we feel that by pushing patients into further suffering, we're taking care of them.

The desire to do "everything" is natural, but all of us—doctors, patients and family members—should consider the other side: Doing everything possible to provide comfort is also a good thing.

Conflicts within the Family

In situations of stress, conflicts are common. In fact, crises such as serious illness sometimes bring out underlying family issues that have nothing directly to do with the circumstances at hand. Whenever disagreement within a patient's family arises, the medical team should meet with the whole family, including the patient, if feasible, to discuss and re-evaluate the situation and explain the patient's status to all of them. If all the people involved meet with the team together, they will likely have fewer conflicts. Plans can be changed based on the new assessment of the patient's condition without adding interpersonal tension to an already difficult state of affairs.

Conflicts may arise because some in the family feel that treatments should not have been started in the first place. If the patient's condition were to improve, that would be great, but conflicts may persist nonetheless. Discussions within the family and with the medical providers will help to bring the whole family together. Often it is the spouse who suffers the most. When the patient dies after enduring the effects of the futile treatments, the spouse may have strong regrets and may even be blamed by other members of the family for causing pain. At such times, the spouse needs support, not blame.

Grief counseling is available at most medical facilities and can help reduce the conflict and guilt associated with any death, especially if the death was painful. If the decision to continue treatment was made after due deliberation and analysis, there is likely to be less regret and conflict.

Medical Bills You May Need to Pay (Co-pays and Deductibles)

Even if you have insurance or other forms of coverage, typically there are co-pays and deductibles for which you as a family are responsible. Keep this in mind when deciding if it is appropriate to put a financial strain on your family for a dubious or limited prolongation of life. Many families have to cut back on essentials like food to pay for treatments.

Co-pays and deductibles vary from plan to plan. Some insurance plans also have a lifetime cap or a cap for a specific incident or occurrence of an illness. In some cases, the direct financial responsibilities of the patient and family can reach tens of thousands of dollars. Treatment in the ICU is usually charged at $10,000 per day and may or may not be fully covered by insurance, depending on the type of plan you have.

With changing rules of insurance and payments for medical treatments, premiums are going up, the amount paid by the insurance companies and the government is declining and the burden on the patient and the family is increasing.

As mentioned earlier, the most common cause of personal bankruptcy in this country is medical bills. Many say that you cannot and should not place a dollar value on the life of a person. But reality has to be faced. If large debts are incurred just to keep someone on life support for a few days, is it fair to the rest of the family? Going into debt is justified if the patient will recover and enjoy a good life. The situations we are discussing do not fall into that category. We are talking about illnesses that are already advanced and for which doctors have made a clear assessment that further treatment will not benefit the patient. In those situations, one must think of the long-term consequences for the rest of the family. Regardless of the outcome, the doctors and hospitals will expect to and will get paid for all the treatments they provide.

Long-term Recovery and Stress on Caregivers

The consequences of undertaking last-ditch treatments last a long time. Even if the treatment has some effect, the patient will not return to good health, even to the health she had before the long-shot treatment was undertaken. There will be an extended period of slow recovery, and the degree of recovery cannot be predicted.

If a patient with emphysema or chronic heart failure develops severe pneumonia that does not respond to standard treatments and the pneumonia advances to the point of requiring life support, recovery is unlikely. Even if the patient survives, there will be further damage to the heart and lungs from the acute stress and infection. The patient will be in a worse state than before the acute insult and may need to go to a rehabilitation center or a skilled nursing facility. During this slow recovery, partial as it will be, the patient and family will continue to suffer.

The family will have a period of months or even years when one or more persons will have to put their lives on hold. If the main caregiver is frail or elderly or has medical problems of his own (not an uncommon situation), the burden can be great and may even cause the caregiver's health to deteriorate. An intervention that produces long-term discomfort and pain should not be undertaken lightly. All pros and cons need to be considered.

When you undertake a treatment that your doctor has told you is not likely to help, the reasons that she recommended not taking it were probably that it had a small chance of immediate control, significant chance of long-term disability and the probability that you would die from the disease anyway. Think about these issues before forcing doctors to give you treatments they do not want to give.

During the long recovery, the stress on the family, particularly on the spouse, who is usually the main caregiver, is great and prolonged. It has been observed that compassion has limits; it can exhaust the caregiver—she can do only so much. Frustrated and angry at their own dependency, some patients lash out at those closest to them. At an emotional level, even though they love the patient, many caregivers often start thinking, "When will this end? How long can I go on like this?" In her book *Knocking on Heaven's Door*, Katy Butler says of her terminally ill father, "I wanted him to die because I loved him."[12]

In our country, many people have limited and restricted insurance coverage. Many do not have insurance because they could not afford the premiums. There are poor and even middle-income people who do not have resources that can be used for long-term care. Think of a family where the children or the spouse need to work without a break to maintain the family income and keep the family together. If they have to take care of someone who is not going to recover, the family can be hurt in many ways. The physical and emotional stress on those who have to take care of someone who will not get better can be severe. The financial burden can ruin the family. Sometimes this is unavoidable, as when a physically healthy person has Alzheimer's disease, but all too often the harm to the family arises because the patient insisted on a treatment that the doctor said was not in his best interest.

As stated above, after certain illnesses, in some cases rehabilitation specialists can restore function and speed up recovery. However, before a rehabilitation program is embarked upon, a proper evaluation and analysis should be undertaken. The parameters to consider are whether the chances of recovery of function are good or poor, whether the patient's general health is good enough to tolerate the rigors of the rehabilitation process (which can be as demanding as strenuous athletic training), and whether or not the underlying disease is going to be cured or put into remission. If a patient has hardening of the arteries (atherosclerosis) in the brain, heart and limbs, she is unlikely to tolerate or benefit from rehabilitation efforts. If the patient has dementia, he will not be able to understand and cooperate with the physical therapist's instructions following a hip replacement, and whatever happens with the new hip, the dementia will continue to get worse.

Actor Christopher Reeve's 1995 fall resulting in the complete severing of his spinal cord was tragic.[13] Most famous for playing Superman, he was at the prime of his life and in excellent health when he fell off his horse, became paralyzed in all four limbs and was unable to breathe on his own. Although it was clear to the physicians and medical scientists that he could not recover, he tried some new and innovative treatments that did not mend his spinal cord. However, he was able to live nine more years, and even to direct films, using a motorized wheelchair and a ventilator. Reeve also established a foundation to fund research into spinal-cord injuries.

Most people are not in a position to undergo rounds of experimental treatments. Reeve could because he was a wealthy celebrity and had been in top physical shape prior to his accident; so he presumably was a good candidate for experimental therapies. For ordinary people, an injury of that nature would have a serious practical, including financial, impact on their families.

Another aspect of long-term rehabilitation has recently emerged. Medicare and the federal government have started funding long-term rehabilitation efforts. This service is unfortunately being misused, occasionally fraudulently. Patients with no potential for improvement in function are being sent to rehabilitation centers—in some cases, only because the facility can make extra money. Some of these places do not have adequate equipment or personnel. They are just in it to get paid.[14]

Katy Butler put it this way: "His stroke devastated two lives. . . . After the stroke, [my mother] cared for my father the way she'd cared for my brothers and me when we were three or four."[15] Butler describes how her mother, who was in her eighties, suffered many health problems while taking care of her elderly, demented, frail husband. Butler's mother did her best but suffered. The tragedy was that the husband had no chance of recovery. He was alive because he got treatments that kept him alive but did not make him better.

As mentioned earlier, a transfer to a rehabilitation facility does not relieve the stress on the family. Rehabilitation is effective in people with one specific problem, like learning to walk or speak after a stroke. In patients with multiple problems that cannot be fixed, rehabilitation just delays the transition to comfort care.

Uncertainty

Throughout a treatment undertaken based on a false hope, there will be a period of uncertainty in which the family just has to wait to see what happens. The family will be in limbo, sometimes for quite awhile. Because doctors are inclined to conduct more treatments rather than less, the patient and family will be better off listening if the doctor recommends stopping the treatments.

Think about the whole picture; take only treatments that have a good chance of meaningful benefit. If you don't, remember who will benefit—the medical system that profits from those treatments. Given all the difficulties you and your family will have to deal with, you will not to come out ahead. In fact, in some fashion, medicine becomes the enemy, and death seems like a friend.

How to Reduce Over-Treatment and Proceed Toward Comfort

As explained in previous chapters, the reasons doctors push treatments are many and varied. Changing a system and the practices of many generations is not going to be easy. Because large numbers of patients are affected by the actions of doctors, some effort must be made to reduce treatments that do not benefit the patient. It would be ideal if the system could be changed. However, if you as a patient understand the whole scenario and the reasons behind the actions of doctors, you can at least exercise more control over your own treatment. Remember, most doctors believe that more treatments are better. It is a part of their mind-set that they must try everything available to them, use technology to the limit and refuse to give up in their effort to defeat your disease.

Pushing treatments is reinforced by doctors' sense of competitiveness, which is especially strong in those who specialize. They look at some parts of the patient's problems and do not place enough importance on the person as whole. Successfully changing the mind-sets of generations of doctors will take systematic re-training and re-education, and it will require time.

In the meanwhile, you should take responsibility for your life, your illness and your death. You should get clear answers regarding the risks and potential benefits of the treatments suggested by your doctor. Some reasons for pushing treatments are related to politics, religion and law. These are big issues, not easy to fix, which need to be tackled by our society because the impact of excessive medical treatments is being felt in the overall economy of the country. It is estimated that the cost of "wasteful" medical treatment in the United States amounted to twice the entire debt of Greece, which caused the euro crisis in 2015.

The American medical system is based on fee-for-service; doctors, hospitals, imaging facilities and laboratories are paid for what they do. Doctors get paid for the treatments they conduct or prescribe; hospitals get paid for each patient who comes to them; imaging facilities and laboratories get paid for each study or test they perform. This creates an incentive for them to do more, because doing more brings in more money. There is no reason for them to reduce treatments. In most cases, doctors are honest and do what they think is needed. But they do not think, "Can I do without this test? Can I do without this treatment without harming the patient?" These unnecessary procedures lead to waste and in some cases harm. The only exceptions are US military and Veterans Administration hospitals and clinics, where they have no financial incentive to do too much.

Teneille Brown, a lawyer I have quoted elsewhere in this book, has extensively reviewed and written about how the payment system for health care gives incentives to oncologists to use more chemotherapy and other aggressive treatments on cancer patients even though it is clear from the beginning that these treatments are unlikely to improve quality of life or prolong it.[1] She points out that the market for chemotherapy is unique in its payment system, which provides incentives to deny death. Oncologists benefit directly from the sale of chemotherapy drugs. Oncologists make more money from chemotherapy than from meeting with patients and reviewing their care. Medicare reimbursement for chemotherapy encourages aggressive treatments. Chemotherapy drugs are not subject to the cost-benefit control and other cost-saving measures that Medicare applies to other drugs. This leads to more expensive drugs being prescribed, even when less costly drugs are equally effective.

Brown's statements have been confirmed by oncologist Laura Tenner and medical ethicist Paul Helft, both physicians themselves.[2] Between 2008 and 2013 the amount spent on anticancer medications globally rose from $71 billion to $95 billion; in other words, it increased by 5 percent every year. Yet the median survival rate for cancer patients increased by only 2.1 months over that period. Tenner and Helft explain one of the reasons behind this as follows: "Because healthcare does not fall under the influence of free market forces, the competition of similar products flooding the market has done nothing to drop the price of these agents."[3]

These negative and positive incentives, which continue to be supported by Congress because of the organized lobbying methods described earlier in this book, lead to over-treatment. In the process, less importance is given to patient care and comfort.

Our system stands in contrast to those of other advanced countries like Canada, Norway, Sweden, Denmark, France, Germany and Great Britain, to name the most obvious ones. In these countries, doctors are paid a salary, so they have no incentive to conduct excessive tests or treatments. They do what is needed. The reality is that the overall cost of medical care in these countries is about half of what it is in the United States—about 10 percent of their gross domestic products compared to 18 percent here. Most importantly, these countries have greater life expectancy and lower infant mortality rates than the United States, a far better index of good health care than money spent. We spend more, and our results are worse. Atul Gawande has discussed this discrepancy in the *New Yorker* in an article titled "The Cost Conundrum."[4]

One relatively simple change in the system would be to provide more support to the families of sick people. If more time and effort is given to explain the situation, they will be able to make informed decisions. The system could provide incentives for medical professionals to conduct such discussions and make time for them.

Attempts are being made to change our country's system, but vested interests, lobbying and politics are making it difficult. The issues are huge. As a patient, you may not be able to reform American medicine; however, being aware of how the system works will help you and your family. Again, asking questions about your own disease and options will protect you from excessive tests and treatment.

Brown has some very useful suggestions that could help reduce some excess in the treatment of cancer and could also help in other areas.[5] These are as follows:

a. Respect provider autonomy and allow, after due discussion, providers to override unreasonable demands from patients and families.
b. Have Medicare and insurance companies pay for discussion of options and end-of-life choices and for providing comfort care that does not entail active treatment of the disease.

c. Reduce payments for procedures and active treatments in the time frame close to death unless there is some specific reason.
d. Through patient and family surveys, find out if patients understand the reason for the treatment. If patients do not understand the goal of the treatment, this suggests that there was poor communication by the doctor. It also suggests that the patient agreed to a treatment without knowing its risks and benefits. Such a procedure may be compensated at a lower rate.
e. Remove incentives for treatment, such as mark-ups for chemotherapy drugs and placement of heart pacemakers.

I understand that these suggestions will be difficult to implement and that defining the limits will be questioned by those with vested interests. In fact, many lobby groups will resist this initiative. But these recommendations will send an important message, and reasonable people will support these measures to provide more comfort and save precious resources.

During the 2008 presidential election, there was a discussion about paying doctors for the time they spent discussing with their patients what they wanted for themselves when they had a serious life-threatening illness. They were encouraged to think of their own advance directives. The doctors were *asked* and encouraged to think what *they* would want in that situation. Vice presidential candidate Sarah Palin labeled such discussions "death panels."[6] This rallied a segment of the population who believed that reformers were "trying to pull the plug on Grandma"—a reference to discontinuing life support. Putting such a negative spin on this simple proposal for reform had a political impact. This was sad, because it sent the message to some that the administration was encouraging doctors to withhold treatments. In reality, it was an attempt to encourage patients and doctors to think about and discuss what was best for the patient.

Another difficult problem is the fear of lawsuits. As discussed earlier in this book, this fear leads to a lot of wasteful tests and treatments. Attempts are being made to improve the relationship between the medical establishment and the legal system. These are small beginnings, but they, too, are being opposed by some vested interests. Most people agree that there are wasteful and excessive treatments and that discouraging them should not open doctors and hospitals to charges of malpractice, but there is little agreement on what to do about it.

Brown has analyzed the situation very carefully. She points out, "While providers fear criminal liability, this is *exceedingly* unlikely. There is no state that criminally prohibits a provider from withdrawing care that is deemed medically ineffective or futile. It does not meet the criminal definition of battery. It is not murder. It is not criminal neglect. As long as the providers are honest with the family about why they are withdrawing care, there is no fraud."[7]

As of now, the best that you as a patient can do is to ask questions and be sure that you are not subjected to unnecessary treatments or tests.

The word "comfort" is used in many ways and sometimes means different things to different people. "I am comfortable saying this" and "I am comfortable making this decision" are just two examples of using the word differently from the way I have used it throughout this book. A doctor certainly might say, "I am not comfortable telling a patient that there are no further treatments available and that comfort care is the best option." Sometimes the word is used very specifically, as when a hospital patient asks the nurse to raise the head of the bed to a more comfortable position.

Even in the context of how you feel during your illness, during its treatment and in the time before your death, there are different ways in which the word "comfort" is commonly used.

To begin with, one person may say, "I am comfortable taking this treatment even though I know it has a small chance of helping me." Another may say, "I want to be comfortable before I die." Focusing on the word as used when we talk about the time before death, there are many senses of "comfortable." Being free of distressing symptoms is one broad category. There are many symptoms that can make you uncomfortable. Pain is probably the most common. (Here again "pain" is used differently in different situations. "So and so is a pain in the neck" is a common metaphorical use.) Shortness of breath, bowel problems, nausea and vomiting are other familiar examples of *dis*comfort. Fever is another symptom that can be distressing. Being free of these symptoms is a part of being comfortable. Not worrying about what may happen is also comforting. Acceptance of what is going to happen is a part of being comfortable. Freedom from fear of financial problems is a part of being comfortable. It is comforting to know that your family and friends will not be devastated by your death. Talking to them freely and openly is a way of getting and providing comfort.

On the other hand, some patients opt for ICU treatments. The idea of receiving aggressive care may initially make them comfortable on an emotional or even ideological level. However, if they and their families consider the other, less abstract senses of "comfort," they may recognize that the reality is very different.

Let us look more specifically and compare some of the treatments that may be used as death approaches and how they contrast with what you can do to make yourself *comfortable*. In the ICU, you will need to be on monitors that will record your heart rate, blood pressure and how much oxygen your body is getting. Monitors are electric devices that are connected to your body either by an electric pad or put into your artery or vein. Most monitors have a light and beeper that flash or beep when your heart rate or the other various parameters they are measuring go above or below a set level. The monitors are essential to letting the medical personnel know the condition of your body, but the beeping and flashing is not conducive to your rest and comfort. Then, of course, if there is a change, the nurses and doctors have to come in and take corrective action. If the treatment in the ICU has a reasonable chance of making you better, this discomfort is justified and appropriate. A detailed and honest discussion with your doctor will be necessary for you to understand the benefits and chances of recovery. If it is just to placate a hope, treatment in the ICU will only make your life difficult.

In case your heart stops beating and you have chosen to have CPR, the process and procedures the doctors and nurses have to undertake to restore the heartbeat are extremely painful; some call them brutal. The heart needs to be brought back to normal, rhythmic beating. This requires either electric shocks to the heart or a large amount of mechanical pressure on the heart, which requires compressing the chest wall and ribs. It is quite common that some ribs are broken because of the chest compression. At the same time, in order to provide adequate amounts of oxygen to the body, a tube has to be inserted into your windpipe (trachea), which is painful. Then oxygen is pushed into your lungs under pressure. If this is likely to restore your body to a functioning status for a reasonable amount of time, it may be worthwhile to suffer through that pain. But, as stated earlier, if the chance is less than 10 percent that you will survive a month and less than 3 percent that you will be reasonably functional, is it worth it?

Treatment in the ICU and CPR most often deprives you of a chance to be comfortable with no benefit despite the pain of the procedures.

Chronic heart and lung diseases are a common cause of death. In the early stages, treatments can be quite effective, especially if the patients follow the prescribed regimen of drugs, weight control and exercise and do not smoke. But the time does come when these measures cease to work and heart and lung function continues to get worse. The patient suffers from shortness of breath, fluid buildup and general weakness. Doctors continue to help the person as well as they can, but the condition deteriorates nonetheless. The patient requires frequent visits to the clinic and needs hospitalization to help control the exacerbation of the chronic problem. He has no life except one relating to his failing organs and attempts to help control the symptoms. Often there is no clear indication of how long the individual can live in that state. Similar situations are faced by patients with chronic liver failure.

Transplantation of the affected organs can help in some cases, especially when the patient is otherwise healthy. This requires an evaluation by specially trained experts. An evaluation, detailed explanation and open discussion with an appropriate specialist may provide valuable information and help.

For some varieties of heart disease, a left ventricular assist device (LVAD) may provide temporary support. This is a very complicated and high-tech apparatus. It is connected to the biggest part of the heart, the left ventricle, and pumps blood into the main artery (the aorta), which carries blood to the whole body. When the left ventricle is unable to pump adequate amounts of blood into the aorta, the LVAD can do that. However, installing the LVAD is a major surgical procedure. This device was designed for short-term use and for patients who have an acute problem, in the hope of tiding them over a crisis. It has also proved helpful for patients who have a good chance of benefiting from a heart transplant and are waiting for a suitable donated organ.

Gradually, the LVAD started being used as a long-term treatment for patients who had chronic left ventricular failure and were not suitable for heart transplantation. It became a "destination treatment," meaning it was to be used until the patient died. According to an article in the August 3, 2015, *Washington Post*, an estimated 250,000 to 300,000 people are now considered candidates for LVAD as a destination treatment.[8]

If the LVAD were a simple device that kept the patient comfortable and if it were easy to manage, using it in patients with chronic left ventricular failure would be worthwhile—but it is not. The article cited above goes on to describe a LVAD recipient who mostly spent his time sitting in a chair unable to participate in any meaningful activities. His wife expended two to three hours a day just changing dressings and taking care of the tubes inserted into his heart. She had little time to do anything else. Despite her efforts, the device got infected and had to be replaced twice; the patient is on his third LVAD. He has had many other medical problems related to the device: bleeding from the stomach and intestine, low blood counts requiring transfusions, and multiple infections. The device has not given the patient or his wife any comfort or quality of life. They now question their decision to agree to the placement of the LVAD.

Their decision was based on hope. Perhaps the doctors had not discussed the option of comfort care as an alternative.

If the function of major organs continues to get worse, consideration needs to be given to changing the goal to comfort and to discontinuing futile attempts to fix the problem. The decision to stop treatments aimed at improving the function of the heart, lung or liver is difficult, but if you find yourself faced with major organ failure, you must talk to your doctors to find out when the emphasis should change to measures that produce more comfort, even if this may shorten the total duration of your life.

Kidney dialysis is an effective procedure to correct some changes in the body's fluid balance and to remove toxic metabolic products. This saves lives if the kidney damage is acute and short term. It can also keep people alive until they get a kidney transplant if that is appropriate. Dialysis may be very helpful, under certain circumstances, in providing benefit to seriously ill patients. Although dialysis is expensive, Medicare covers it fully for individuals with end-stage renal disease.

However, if the kidney damage is permanent and patients have chronic problems like heart and lung damage, advanced diabetes (one of the most common causes of kidney failure) with damage to multiple organs, or mental deterioration, dialysis will be needed for the rest of their lives as they suffer from the effects of their other illnesses.

To be truly effective, long-term dialysis requires regular treatments that vary from three times per week to daily. Each dialysis treatment generally necessitates a minimum of three to four hours to be optimally effective. Patients must incorporate dramatic changes to their lifestyles that include dietary and fluid restrictions and highly regimented medication schedules. These changes are often very difficult for patients to make and may dramatically alter their quality of life and their overall perceived comfort or well-being. For some, the dialysis treatments represent a recurring uncomfortable, unpleasant experience. Most individuals who require extended dialysis do not recover enough kidney function to maintain a life independent of dialysis. Most associated medical problems usually keep getting worse, and the patient's quality of life and overall well-being progressively diminish.

Unfortunately, many end-stage kidney patients also have heart and lung problems; so even on the days they are not getting the dialysis, they are not very functional. If the patient has chronic debility or mental deterioration, she can be kept alive with the use of dialysis, but the individual and her family members need at least to ask whether she is getting any benefit. If dialysis is stopped after considering all the advantages and disadvantages to the patient, she can die comfortably in a week or so without suffering. As before, I am not advocating for or against dialysis but do feel it important that every end-stage kidney patient ask the question.

For many advanced cancer patients, comfort during the last stages of the disease is the goal. This means having a life with minimal problems from pain, bowel issues, nausea and vomiting. For many cancer patients, it also means being in familiar, calm surroundings and interacting with people they love. It is possible to provide these to most patients. The best setting to achieve these comfort goals is at home, with hospice professionals assisting the patient and family.

In the September 2015 issue of *JAMA Oncology*, Charles Blanke and Erik Fromme suggested that for patients with cancer who are likely to die in the next six months, the default action should be *no active treatment*. This means that unless there is some clear and compelling reason to give chemotherapy, comfort measures and care should be provided instead.[9]

If the decision is made to "try one more treatment," the goal of comfort is more difficult to reach. Taking another treatment requires that the patient makes visits to the hospital or clinic. Blood tests and X-rays are necessary. Then the patient has to deal with the side effects of the chemotherapy. One needs to look at the pros and cons and decide whether the best results will come from comfort care or from active treatment.

Comfort, pain-free life with family and friends in familiar surroundings can be most effectively achieved if we recognize the limits of medicine and accept what is most likely to happen. Comfort before death can be provided and achieved in almost all situations—once comfort is accepted as a goal. It is one of the best gifts we can give to ourselves and to our loved ones.

When you are faced with a situation in which the treatment for your disease did not help you, obtaining more information is the next step. You need to put together the information that you have collected regarding the status of your disease, the previous treatments and the options at the present time. Match these with your values and goals. Also discuss them with those you are close to and trust.

If in your analysis, further treatment of the disease does not fit with your values and goals, you have other options—the option to choose care over treatment. They are not the same.

Once you accept that active treatment of your disease is not in your best interest, there are other methods for dealing with the admittedly sad situation and prevent it from getting worse. Broadly there are three ways to approach this, and they are all directed toward comfort before death. Remember, the goal is comfort. The goal is not control of your disease. Changing your goal to comfort allows you and your family to be together.

The three approaches are not mutually exclusive; they can be combined and utilized as needed. Which of these you use and when is up to you and is dependent on your condition, on the nature and extent of the disease and on the circumstances as they change. The process is a continuum, so different approaches are helpful at different points, until the time of death.

The broad categories of these measures are as follows:

a. Comfort care
   i. Control of symptoms
   ii. Hospice
b. Hastening death by passive methods
c. Hastening death by active means

COMFORT CARE

As a patient, you have the right to choose the option of being comfortable and making the best of your time with your family and friends. You can choose not to take certain drugs and not to undergo surgery, dialysis or treatment in the ICU. At any point in the course of the illness, you can refuse any treatment.

The decision should, of course, be made after full analysis of the benefits and risks involved.

If you choose to stop taking active treatments for your advanced disease and to receive comfort care instead, your chances of being comfortable and spending quality time with your family and friends are good. You can enjoy the people who matter to you most for whatever time you have. Most likely you will have no regrets, and your family will be happy to give you the care you require.

When you make a conscious decision to face death on your own terms, you get a tremendous amount of personal power. After analyzing the information received from your doctor, and after discussing it with your family and friends, you can refuse further treatment aimed at controlling your disease. Refusal is not "suicide." You should make the decision on the basis of your values and what is important to you. If you still have the energy, you may decide to visit one of the places on your "bucket list" or to return to your childhood vacation spot on the coast. A friend of mine knew a woman with Stage IV breast cancer who chose two weeks in Paris over yet another round of chemotherapy.

The most common reason for patients to refuse treatments, when the chances of benefit are small, is that, like most people, they value comfort and quality of life. They feel that a small improvement in their condition is not worth the risks, pain and discomfort of the treatment.

Control of Symptoms

Once you have made the decision not to undertake active treatments, you can focus on being comfortable. Your medical providers should and will work with you to supply you with one or more of the tools to give you a comfortable life. Palliative medical care and hospice are two commonly used approaches. They have a common goal—your comfort. They work together and with you and your family in a coordinated manner. Depending on your needs, your family and your home situation, you can be in your home or in a hospice, a specialized care facility for patients nearing the end of life who prefer not to be at home.

The term "palliative" is used in many different ways depending on the situation and also on who is using it. *Webster's Dictionary* defines its medical meaning as "something that reduces the effects or symptoms of a medical condition without curing it."[10] In the medical context, one use of the term "palliative care" is an active treatment given to help relieve a symptom or problem without expectation of curing the patient. Take, for example, a patient who has a large cancerous mass pressing on a vital structure. The nature of the cancer is such that the disease cannot be eradicated. But chemotherapy, surgery or radiation therapy could take the pressure off that vital structure and make the patient feel better. Such approaches prompted the use of the word "palliative" to describe any treatment expected to give at least partial relief. In some cases palliative care specialists work with patients who do not have a terminal illness but have symptoms that their other doctors are not able to control—for example, pain from chronic neurological disorders.

Unfortunately, it has become more and more common to treat a cancerous lesion "because it is there," meaning that the doctor knows that none of the techniques prescribed will cure the cancer. Even if patients have no symptoms from the cancer, doctors often will treat them with no specific goal or aim. Thus, chemotherapy is now being given to more and more cancer patients. Worse still, the chemotherapy is being given for longer periods and at a time close to death. This is also referred to as "palliative treatment," misleadingly, even though nothing is being palliated.

This leads to a poorer quality of life for patients in the time preceding death and does not prolong life. This approach has been questioned by some but continues in many oncology settings.[11]

This problem has been carefully analyzed by sociologist Isabelle Baszanger, as well as by attorney and medical ethicist Teneille Brown.[12] They agree that the practice of administering such active treatments when cancer patients are near death should be reduced, so that patients will have more comfort at life's end.

In surveys, when doctors were asked if they had an irreversible brain injury, what procedures or treatments would they like to have done on themselves, most of them stated that they would not want active treatments. For example, 60 percent would not want intravenous fluids or antibiotics. Eighty to ninety percent would not want surgery, dialysis or CPR. They would like to die comfortably and in peace.[13]

All physicians have knowledge of drugs and procedures that can be used to relieve a patient's symptoms. Palliative care physicians are specialists who have extra training that enables them to relieve certain symptoms that may not have been controlled by other physicians' efforts. Pain is one of the symptoms that afflict many people with uncontrollable disease. But there are other symptoms, not just physical pain, that affect some people. Sometimes the word "suffering" is used. The discussion of pain and suffering is complex, and philosophers have addressed the issue at length for millennia. This is not the place for a philosophical discussion. Instead, I will address some of the symptoms that are common when disease progresses or organs are not working normally. These symptoms are easily controlled in most people but may be difficult to relieve in some. With their specialized training, palliative care physicians can often help control symptoms.

Physical pain can result from different problems—growth of tumors in different organs, damage to bones and pressure on nerves, to name a few. The treatment depends on the cause of the pain. Apart from pain medications, there may be methods for removing that cause. For example, sometimes radiation is utilized to relieve the pressure on nerves.

The most important point is that pain is something the *patient* feels; no one else can feel it. The approach, therefore, is to give the right type of pain medication in adequate amounts. There is no fixed or defined dose. The patient should receive as much pain medication as needed to relieve the pain. The limitation is that pain medications can cause side effects. Some of these, such as constipation and nausea, are common, and physicians can use other medications to prevent or counter them.

The other common side effect of pain medication is drowsiness and an inability to think clearly. This can present a dilemma, because most people would like to fulfill their lives and interact with family and friends when they are dying. Here again, you as the patient are the one who can decide best. You can increase and decrease the dose of pain medications, especially the morphine-like drugs—opioids. If you prefer, you can cut back on the medication for some period of time to allow you to be more alert when you have visitors or need to deal with matters related to your estate. You may experience some pain as a trade-off for being alert, but you can increase the dosage after your family, friends or advisors are gone. Such adjustments can be made by you depending on your need and desire. The medical team can guide you.

In some cases, especially late in the course of illness when death is near, the pain may be so severe that the only way to control it is to make you drowsy or put you into a drug-induced coma. This method, used as a last resort, has been called "terminal sedation." In this situation, death occurs from the progressive disease, but the patient is not aware. Death may be hastened by complications related to the drug-induced coma, but its intended purpose is to relieve suffering, not to cause death.

Constipation, nausea and stomach- and bowel-related problems can occur because of problems with functions of the stomach or intestines and also because of pain medications. There are many ways to control these symptoms; the treatment depends on the cause of the difficulty.

Shortness of breath can result from problems in the heart or lungs. Most often doctors control these problems by providing additional oxygen to the patient through a small tube placed in the nose or a mask placed over the mouth and nose. If this is not enough, your distress from lack of oxygen can be relieved by morphine. Morphine, in addition to relieving pain, acts on the brain sensors that detect the lack of oxygen. The use of morphine does not improve the oxygen supply to the body, but it does relieve the sense of suffocation. By using enough oxygen and morphine, you can be made comfortable before you die.

As the organs continue to deteriorate and cannot do what they should, fluid can build up in the lungs, abdomen and limbs. This is a sign of a failing body and in itself does not require any treatment. It is a part of the process of death. Another type of fluid buildup occurs in some patients with advanced cancer. This is because the cancer cells invade the covering of the heart, lungs or intestines. The cancer cells cause the lining or covering to secrete fluid, leading to difficulty in breathing or distention of the abdomen. This can be distressing and may require draining the fluid with a needle, which can provide significant comfort. The patient should decide when to drain the liquid.

There are many other problems that can cause distress to the patient before death. All doctors can help alleviate these symptoms by using drugs to relieve them or, if possible, working on the cause of the problem. In some cases, they may need the expertise of palliative care physicians, whose medical specialty is symptom relief. As a part of the process of providing comfort before death, it is also possible to use the services provided by hospice.

Hospice

"Hospice" has two meanings: the facilities and the people who help you and your family in the last months of life and an approach, an idea—the idea that everyone is entitled to comfort before death.

We want our experience of dying to be peaceful and dignified. As family members and friends, we want to know that our loved one was pain-free and comfortable at the time of death. Katy Butler confirms the reports that three out of four people want to die at home, like their ancestors did.[14] Unfortunately, only one out of four do. This is because, for various reasons (discussed elsewhere in this book), they undertake life-sustaining treatments that require being in the hospital; thus, they die there. The mission of the hospice organizations that exist in most American communities is to give terminally ill patients and their families the practical and emotional support they need so that the patients can die comfortably in a place of their choosing.

In India, most people approaching death remain at home, cared for by their family members, who typically live nearby. During a recent trip there, I visited my 88-year-old cousin, Usha di. She had been very weak for a long time. The doctors had conducted blood tests and found that she had kidney failure. They suggested kidney dialysis. Her daughter felt that dialysis would be painful and would not make her feel better. The family declined the dialysis but continued her medications for high blood pressure and tried to give her food and water. This was distressing to my cousin.

During my visit, Usha di recognized me, and we talked briefly about old times, but she could not be very interactive.

We had a family meeting. I suggested that the medication be stopped, and the family agreed. I further recommended that we stop insisting on feeding her and that we not give her water unless she asked for it. My cousin's daughter, a mature and thoughtful woman, said she would need to think about that. After a day or so, she agreed that forcing water was just causing her mother distress. The family made sure that someone was always with my cousin. Someone was there to touch her, rub her hands and forehead and make sure she was comfortable. She gradually slipped into a coma. After about 10 days, my niece called, asking, "How long can this go on?" I assured her that Usha di was in no distress and that we should continue to keep her peaceful. She died two days later. The family donated her eyes to the eye bank to restore vision to a blind person. They also donated her body for medical research.

The family had closure. They had the reassurance that my cousin did not suffer. They had the satisfaction that, even in death, Usha di helped other people.

In America, where many people do not have extended family nearby, hospice delivers services that allow them to receive comfort care at home.

There are hospice organizations in most cities around the country. They work with different hospitals and doctors to provide practical and emotional support for patients who have a terminal illness and want to die in comfort. When the patient, the family and the doctors agree that the best way to help the patient is to stop attempts at treating the disease and work toward comfort, hospice can get involved.

In some situations, if the needs of the patient are such that family members are not able to take care of them, hospice support can be provided in assisted-living facilities, nursing homes or even hospitals.

Goals for comfort are worked out between the patient and the medical providers. Hospice professionals (typically registered nurses) determine what is bothering the patient and help formulate a plan to control the symptoms. The hospice team discusses this with the patient and the patient's physicians, and the details are worked out. The ideal is that the patient will be able to go home, and the comfort measures will be implemented there. As the end of life nears, the patient can be in a familiar environment with family and friends.

Apart from the medications and other medical requirements, hospice also takes care of day-to-day needs. If you require a special bed to make it easier to sit up, that is arranged. If your mobility is limited, arrangements are made for a walker or a bedside commode. After you are home, members of the hospice team are available to help you and your caregivers. They arrange for refills of medications and for special diets. If you ever experience sudden distress, doctors and nurses can still help with that. The members of the hospice team are always available to help the family with medical and emotional support. They also have trained personnel who can provide bereavement counseling.

Hospice also helps avoid a panic call to 911, which a family member may make if, for example, the patient is struggling for breath. Instead, the hospice team can arrive at the patient's home promptly to reassure the caregivers and to provide relief of the acute distress. A call to 911 for a patient who is dying compounds the tragedy, because emergency responders are required by law to deal with the immediate issue. They cannot take the patient's terminal illness into account, thus defeating the very purpose of comfort before death. They even have to try CPR immediately if the patient's heart has stopped.

There is a provision in most states for physicians to complete and sign an Emergency Medical Service—Do Not Resuscitate (EMS-DNR) form. This gives explicit orders to the emergency medical service personnel not to attempt CPR on a terminally ill patient. The EMS-DNR form must be presented to the team responding to the 911 call. It is a doctor's order and must be followed. The EMTs have to provide other means to relieve the patient's distress. But if the family does not have that order in hand (clipping it to the door of the refrigerator, rather than, say, sticking it in a file cabinet, is a good idea), the EMTs are obligated to do everything possible to try to revive the patient. Remember, in most cities the emergency medical service is part of the fire department. These dedicated and often heroic men and women are trained to act—to save the patient's life, right then, no matter how painful and futile the method may be. Calling 911 puts this all-out effort in motion.

Once comfort is agreed upon as the goal, hospice, the patient's doctor and the doctors from hospice all work together. Many doctors who work for hospice organizations have training in palliative care. The roles of the patient's own doctors, the palliative care doctors and the hospice doctors are a continuum. Depending on the circumstances, one or more of them may be needed to provide the best care and comfort to the patient. They also form a pyramid. Most people can be made comfortable with relatively simple measures. Some require the help of those with more specialized training. In certain circumstances, measures described in the next section may be needed to reduce the duration of a patient's suffering. The pyramid means that only a few people need the help of a specialist and only rarely does a patient need to hasten death. But that option is comforting to many patients and family members.

A woman whose husband had died said, "Because of the support he received, my husband died well. Because my husband died well, I live well." Some studies have reported that patients with advanced lung cancer lived longer when they were on hospice with comfort care than those who received chemotherapy. Also, they had a better quality of life.[15]

Here is an experience related to me by a young medical student. This story and many like it show the benefits of comfort care rather than continued, futile treatment of the disease. A painful death with problems related to the treatment is not the only way to die. Jasmine Nanez describes an elderly veteran who did not want more treatment and wanted to die in peace:

At the VA I had a certain patient who reminded me so much of someone I knew. The person I knew was not in his 80s, so that is not where the similarities came from. Instead, I found that my patient made the same sad, grumpy and hopeless faces as the person I used to know. Because of that, I felt this sort of heart break for my patient whenever he was down, which was often. He was in his 80s, his wife had passed away a few years ago, and he really seemed hopeless to me. He was in the VA for treatment for cancer. He was not a surgical candidate, so he was undergoing chemo and radiation therapy. He hated it. It seemed like he was talked into it by his Primary Care Physician (PCP); he was not hopeful that he would get better. He was hopeless and seemed ready to die. He did not see any point in living anymore. His wife was dead, and he was not able to live on his own anymore. His brother had moved all of his stuff out of his cabin and put it into a garage. So he was depressed. Why had he collected all these things in life to just have them stuffed into a garage? The first day I saw him he was cheerful and even made a few jokes. But nearly a week later, he didn't even smile anymore. The treatment was painful, and he didn't have many visitors. He was hard of hearing, so he was quite isolated. One day I finally asked him if he wanted to continue with the therapy. He couldn't hear me, so I wrote it out on a piece of paper. He read it and thought for a minute. And then he said quite emphatically, "No." He did not want to continue with the therapy, even if his pain could be controlled; he was done with it. He hated every minute of it, and he was not going to do it anymore. In fact, he wanted to leave. I felt confused. On the one hand he seemed really happy that I had offered him this option. It was his choice to make and he could stop therapy any time he wanted. On the other hand, I knew he wouldn't survive long. Maybe that's what he wanted. He said he would go live with his brother, but when we spoke to his brother it turned out it really was not an option. His brother's wife had already taken care of two family members on their death beds, and her health was poor; she didn't have it in her to do it again. But if he could be placed [in a hospice], then they would be able to visit him and care for him that way. I wonder what my reaction to the whole ordeal would have been if he had not reminded me so much of someone I knew. Would his pain hurt me so much?

Accepting help from the personnel at hospice is not giving up; it reflects a change in goal. It is getting the best help and services from the appropriate professionals. As my friend Denys Cope, an RN, stated, "Even when there is some acceptance of death, many people feel completely inadequate to deal with the process."[16]

For advanced cancer, it is clear that patients who are sick and have not had a response to previous treatments get no benefit from last-ditch chemotherapy.

They do not live longer, nor do they feel better.[17] This raises the question: Is there a way to determine in advance and to predict which patients have a better chance of benefiting from chemotherapy? The same study found that patients who could perform their activities of daily living with ease had a better chance of at least maintaining that status. Patients who were sicker and could not perform such routine tasks as dressing, showering and fixing a sandwich without help got worse after chemotherapy. This should be a lesson to my colleague who has patients who can barely walk across the clinic to get the chemotherapy he prescribes.

Unfortunately, hospice services are not used to their full extent, and many patients do not get the benefit of what hospice has to offer. Further, referral to hospice is often done late. Even though hospice organizations use as a benchmark that they can be brought in when the patient is expected to live no longer than six months, the average length of time from referral to hospice and death is three weeks. This deprives dying patients of the benefit of comfort for a meaningful time. Medical providers are being educated about the benefits of hospice services, and the use of hospice is increasing, but often it is the family members, who typically need the support of hospice as much as or more than the patient, who resist. They equate calling on hospice to giving up, to admitting that the person they love will not recover. This is regrettable, because the patient's comfort should be the main concern for us all.

HASTENING DEATH BY PASSIVE METHODS

In some situations patients feel that waiting to die is in itself a burden. There are certain symptoms that even the best efforts cannot alleviate, such as severe respiratory compromise that oxygen and morphine are not able to relieve and severe heart failure that cripples the patient. Sometimes the pain may be so extreme that it can be controlled only by making the patient drowsy or even comatose. In these situations, the patient suffers from continuous distress with no hope of relief. Some forms of cancer cause fluid buildup or bowel problems that cannot be relieved. In such circumstances, patients may feel that they would like to shorten the time to death. They see no benefit in waiting to die. In these extreme cases, there are measures that the patient can take to hasten her own death.

One way of hastening death is to stop taking liquids or food. In any case, for patients who are very weak and have advanced disease, the desire for food and water is decreased. Often family members feel they should give food and water to the dying person; it is an expression of love and concern. Many patients eat and drink only because their loved ones urge them to, although they themselves experience no hunger or thirst. Voluntarily stopping eating and drinking is not painful, and it is legal. Of course, if you are thirsty, you should drink, and if you are hungry, you should eat. But if you don't feel the urge, you do not have to do it just to satisfy your family. Without adding to your burden of symptoms, you can shorten the time to your death—which was bound to happen soon anyway.

Refusing feeding tubes, intravenous fluids and dialysis are ways to hasten death passively. These are medical interventions, and patients have the right to refuse them.

There are some physicians who advocate heavy doses of morphine or sedatives. They suggest using the drugs to the point that the patient goes into a drug-induced coma, the terminal sedation mentioned earlier. This does relieve the symptoms, but the family is forced to watch the patient lying helpless and unconscious, and they are not able to interact. Furthermore, the comatose patient is at high risk for pneumonia and other complications that cause fever and worsening of breathing problems. The duration of such a coma cannot be predicted; the patient and the family are in limbo. The coma is said to relieve distress, but it causes other types of distress. Death is hastened indirectly—but hastened nevertheless. This approach has been called the Doctrine of Double Effect and is legally accepted based on a ruling of the US Supreme Court made in the 1990s, as well as by the Catholic Church and other religious groups.[18] The rationale is that the intent of medicating the patient to the point of continuous unconsciousness, even though this may have life-threatening side effects, was not to kill him but to relieve his suffering.

HASTENING DEATH BY ACTIVE MEANS
Hastening one's own death willfully and actively, with the means and relevant information provided by a physician, can also be humane. A method for accomplishing this is currently legal in the United States only in California, Montana, Oregon, Vermont and Washington, and several other states are considering permitting this approach. The key here is that the patient has the option of ending her own life, painlessly and at a time of her choosing. The doctor does not directly intervene—in fact, he/she is not present.

Even the terms used to discuss this option are contentious. In many cases, those opposed to this approach deliberately misuse the terminology to generate confusion or to give the practice a negative, even barbaric, image. Even though the concept is controversial, a recent Huffington Post/YouGov Poll found that more than two-thirds of Americans said that it should be legal for a physician to assist a terminally ill patient in hastening his death if the patient requests this help.[19] Multiple polls indicate that the public support for Aid in Dying (AiD) is growing.[20] Even the prestigious Fred Hutchinson Cancer Center in Seattle supports AiD.[21]

AiD becomes an option when patients who are dying have tried a variety of methods and drugs to relieve their symptoms and have had limited success. They are forced to make the choice between suffering or being sedated to the point that they are unable to interact with their family or even take care of their most basic needs. If, at this point, the patient feels it would be appropriate to have at hand a means of hastening death, such as a prescribed lethal dose of medication, his desires should be accepted legally, ethically and morally.

There are those who oppose this method of comfort at the end of life, which shortens the time of suffering when death is coming soon anyway. These groups, the strongest and most vociferous of which is the Catholic Church, base their opposition on religious and moral grounds. The Council of Catholic Bishops, nationally and through statements citing their doctrine and raising the issue of sanctity of life, has objected to this practice.[22] They state clearly that they cannot accept a procedure where the *intent* is to kill the patient. However, as an extension of this idea, they do support terminal sedation as described above. They say that if a physician puts a patient into a drug-induced coma after trying all other methods to alleviate symptoms and the patient dies as a result of the complications of the coma, this is acceptable because the doctor's *intent* was to relieve pain, not to end the patient's life. The issue has been debated frequently, but no agreement has yet been reached because of strong feeling, rigid posturing and firmly held belief systems. Deliberately turning off a ventilator is also an act where the intention is to kill the patient, but that is apparently acceptable to the church, because the ventilator is an artificial mechanism that can be seen as interfering with the natural process of dying.

What has been accepted legally and by the public in the five states mentioned above is that terminally ill, mentally competent adults should have the right to end their lives at a time of their choosing and that they can enlist medical assistance. The law in those states allows a willing physician to pre-scribe a lethal dose of a drug if the patient asks for it and to tell the patient how to take it effectively. The drug is available to the patient to use at a time of her choosing. Note that doctors are not *required* to give AiD. The physician is free to follow his conscience.

Some people worry that AiD may lead to patients being coerced by fam-ily members or heirs into ending their lives prematurely. These are personal concerns and need to be respected. However, there are safeguards in place in all five states to prevent coercion and misuse. In Oregon, where AiD has been legal for 20 years, there has been no instance of misuse of the law.[23] Each vol-untary death was carefully documented. All patients were terminally ill and chose AiD on their own.

In 2013 in Oregon, 122 people who were dying requested and received the prescription of a lethal dose. Of these, 77 took the medication and died. This comes to 22 deaths with AiD for every 1,000 deaths in the state.[24] Looked at another way, 37 percent of the patients who received lethal prescriptions never used them to end their lives. Apparently, just being aware that they had the option gave them comfort.

Having control over their deaths gives patients assurance that they can end their suffering when they choose. Further, the discussion that led to legaliza-tion of AiD also increased the awareness and use of comfort care, palliative care and hospice in those states as a whole. Even people who thought that AiD was morally wrong began to ask themselves whether requests for it might be due, in part, to the lack of availability or public awareness of comfort care and of practical and emotional support for families with terminally ill members. Improvements in care may be the reason why many filled the prescription but did not use it.

The process available in the five states has been described in different ways by different people and by different organizations. The most important point to understand is that the drug is voluntarily ingested by the patient. The doc-tor only writes the prescription. Therefore, it is *not euthanasia*. Euthanasia is a process whereby the physician or someone else actively administers a drug to a patient or commits another action with the intent of killing. We should note that "euthanasia" is a Greek word coined in the third century BCE. It means "good death." In 1869 William Lecky gave the word its current meaning.[25] If the patient takes the drug voluntarily, it is not euthanasia.

Other terms used in this context are "assisted suicide" and "physician-assisted suicide." These terms are misleading and are not sensitive to the reason for allowing a terminally ill patient to have more control over the time of his death. Suicide is when, for whatever reason, a person who would otherwise not die in the near future chooses death over life. Helping a person to choose death over life actively is assisting suicide. Physician who help terminally ill patients to hasten their rapidly approaching deaths are not helping them to choose death over life. They are helping them to take control of the time of death.

"Physician-assisted suicide" and "physician-assisted death" may be accurate terms in themselves, but they emphasize the wrong part of the process. The term "Aid in Dying" avoids this confusion. This clarifies that the terminally ill patients want to control the means and timing of their own deaths, and the physician "aids" them by prescribing a drug that will end their lives quickly and painlessly and that they can use at a time of their own choosing. Once they have the means, they can choose the time of their deaths. They can say their goodbyes, be with their families and friends and die with them nearby. The family can celebrate the patient's life, and the patient dies peacefully. This scenario occurs openly in the five states where AiD is legal.

An editorial in the July 2, 2014, issue of the thoughtful *British Medical Journal* fully supported what in the United Kingdom is called the Assisted Dying Bill. This piece of legislation was under discussion in Parliament. The journal stated, "Lord Falconer's Assisted Dying Bill is expected to receive its second reading in the House of Lords this month. The BMJ hopes that this Bill will eventually become law."[26] In supporting the bill, the editorial gave as its reasons that it would reduce suffering and give autonomy to the patient, and assisted dying would be voluntary for both the patient and the doctor. Further, like the laws in the five states in the United States, the proposed legislation contained ample safeguards from the hypothetical objections raised by those who opposed it. Another article, this one in the *Journal of the American Medical Association*, also supported legalization of AiD. JAMA stated, "By restricting Aid in Dying to competent and terminally ill adults, the law can ease the dying process for patients and their families, and avoid the potential of the mistreatment of patients."[27]

Lord Falconer's bill was defeated in the British Parliament on September 11, 2015. However, an editorial in another highly respected UK medical journal, the *Lancet*[28] strongly supported the legislation. The editorial also discussed the issue of palliative care physicians opposing the bill. Apparently, a powerful politician who was also a professor of palliative care objected to the bill. Similar objections have also been raised by some prominent palliative care physicians in the United States. Their argument essentially is that they (palliative care specialists) can control all symptoms for all patients and that therefore AiD is not needed. They do not cite any moral objection to AiD. I disagree with that contention. Yes, these specialists do a good job, but there are many patients whose symptoms cannot be relieved, and AiD is the only way to relieve their suffering. The *Lancet* editorial states, "It is true that the majority of doctors whose professional lives are dedicated to caring for the terminally ill are opposed to assisted dying. But palliative care physicians should not have a monopoly on deciding the place of assisted dying in society."[29]

Support for AiD is growing around the world. An article in the British weekly news magazine *The Economist* strongly supports the idea of allowing sick people to end their lives voluntarily at a time of their choosing.[30] The magazine cites surveys from Western Europe and the United States that show that most people support this practice.

Over recent decades, our social attitudes have changed regarding same-sex marriage, women's right to equal treatment in the workplace and other former taboos. A similar shift, I hope, will occur regarding the idea of giving control to patients who are dying and do not want to prolong their suffering. In all these cases, the public needs to recognize that the action is voluntary and carried out after due thought, and that it is a personal choice.

A practice very different from the above occurs regularly in states where AiD is not legal. Patients commit suicide but often do so surreptitiously. They may hoard the pain medications prescribed to them. Then they take the drug quietly on their own, often alone. The family may experience pain and panic if they find their terminally ill loved one unresponsive. Worse, they may call 911 because they did not know the patient's intention. A whole chain of events ensues that defeats the goal of a comfortable death. Dying in this manner is not a good death.

There are other methods that are cruel and can cause more pain than comfort. I was told by a friend of Molly Ivins that when the late columnist's father learned that he had incurable lung cancer, he shot himself with his pistol. Some desperate people put a plastic bag over their heads or breathe helium.

These procedures have to be done without help from anyone. Even if the family is present, they cannot help the patient. Any help by a second person is technically murder, not just assisting in death.

A comfortable death that is voluntary, open and legal is better than the options just discussed.

The benefits and harms of, the acceptance of and opposition to AiD are major topics of discussion and disagreement. Concerned laypeople, health professionals, religious organizations and politicians all participate in the debate, and many have strong opinions on the subject. Most of this book has covered topics that describe how you can make the best decisions for yourselves.

Tom Beauchamp and James Childers of the Kennedy Institute of Ethics at Georgetown University in Washington have created a framework through which ethics in medically related fields can be analyzed.[31] Their framework suggests using four parameters that allow a comprehensive, broad based analysis of difficult ethical questions. These can be applied to individual cases and also to larger issues affecting society. The four are as follows:

1. Autonomy: The principle that independent actions and choices of the individual should not be constrained by others.
2. Beneficence: The principle that one has a duty to help others by doing what is best for them.
3. Non-malfeasance (doing no harm): The principle that one has a duty not to inflict evil, harm or risk of harm on others. (Obviously this principle is related to that of beneficence.)
4. Justice: The principle that the action should be fair to all.

How do these four principles apply to someone who is suffering, has a limited life expectancy and voluntarily wants to end his own life to stop his suffering?

1. Autonomy: The person wants to end his own life. That person should have the freedom and autonomy to do so. There is no coercion. It is a voluntary act.
2. Beneficence: The end of suffering is a great benefit to that person. If suffering is a harm, then ending it is a benefit.

3. Non-malfeasance: There is no harm. To the person who is suffering, death is not a harm. There are those who say that death is always a harm. Well, death is inevitable and thus in itself cannot and should not be seen as a harm. Sanctity of life is a principle that many abide by. What does that mean? Some say it means that one should not take one's own life. If someone is going to die in the near future, does speeding up death violate the sanctity? Yes, taking another person's life is breaking the principle of sanctity of life, but taking control of the time and manner of one's own death is not.

4. Justice: Allowing AiD is fair to the person who is suffering. No one else is involved. No one else is hurt. It is just to all and should be available to any terminally ill, mentally competent adult patient anywhere.

Thus, AiD passes the test of the principles of biomedical ethics, tests which have been accepted for four decades as the best way to judge if action is ethical.

Comfort at death is a goal we all have for ourselves. We should work to make it a reality for everyone by refusing treatments with low chance of benefit, actively seeking palliative treatments and requesting help from hospice when needed. We can hasten the process by voluntarily refusing water and food and, if needed, should have the option of receiving a physician's help in dying.

In addition to AiD, Compassion and Choices is an organization that provides information on a variety of issues related to living well with serious illness, including advance care planning, comfort care and, if needed, information on hastening one's death. They can be reached at 1-800-247-7421 or CompassionAndChoices.org.

This book resulted from years of experience working with patients, talking to families of patients, studying under teachers and then mentoring young students and doctors myself. Medicine changed in many ways between the time I entered medical school in 1953 and my retirement in 2013. The advances in medical technology are obvious and have led to major benefits to almost everyone. Human thinking and attitudes have been slower to change. Many people have not accepted the need to follow the most crucial recent advance in medicine—recognition of the importance of a healthy lifestyle. Smoking remains common, and obesity and lack of exercise harm millions every year. Society and the medical system are trying to rectify the problem.

Another problem, at the other end of the spectrum, also remains. People are slow to accept the reality that advances in medical technology will not eliminate illness and death.

In writing this book, I have tried to provide a perspective at a personal level, addressing what would help *you* when you or your loved one are seriously ill or facing death. I have attempted to provide a look into some of what may happen and how you can come out ahead in the face of a difficult situation.

I have not attempted to sway you or to tell you how to act or even what decisions to make. I hope that a broad understanding of the actions and motives of all involved will give you a better grasp of this reality: *Nobody gets out of here alive.*

In considering how to live well with serious illness, it is worthwhile to remember the "Serenity Prayer" by the American theologian Reinhold Niebuhr:

God, grant us the serenity to accept the things we cannot change;
Courage to change the things we can;
And wisdom to know the difference.[32]

This will give you a chance to have a good death. A death that is not painful. A death that is accepted by you and by those around you. A death that gives you and your loved ones an opportunity to celebrate your life.

Notes

INTRODUCTION

1. Nick Turse, "For America, Life Was Cheap in Vietnam," *The New York Times* (October 9, 2013), http://www.nytimes.com/2013/10/10/opinion/for-america-life-was-cheap-in-vietnam.html.

2. Joan Halifax, "Compassion and the True Meaning of Empathy," TED, posted September 2011, https://www.ted.com/talks/joan_halifax/transcript?language=en.

CHAPTER 1

1. Sacred Texts, "The Mustard Seed," http://www.sacredtexts.com/bud/btg/btg85.htm.

2. Elisabeth Kübler-Ross, *On Death and Dying* (New York: MacMillan, 1969).

3. Daniel Callahan, *What Kind of Life* (New York: Simon and Schuster, 1991).

4. Sherwin B. Nuland, *How We Die: Reflections on Life's Final Chapter* (New York: Vintage Books, 1993).

CHAPTER 2

1. National Cancer Institute, "Milestone (1971): National Cancer Act of 1971," https://dtp.cancer.gov/timeline/flash/milestone/M4_Nixon.htm.

2. H. K. Koh, "The Arc of Health Literacy," *Journal of the American Medical Association* 314, no. 12 (September 22/29, 2015): 1225.

3. Barry Furrow et al., *Bioethics: Healthcare Law and Ethics*, 7th ed. (St. Paul: West Academic Publishing, 2013), 324–25.

4. Ibid., 403.

5. Teneille Brown, "Denying Death," *Arizona Law Review* 56, no. 4 (2015): 22.

6. Stephanie Armour, "End-of-Life Discussions Will Be Reimbursed by Medicare," *Wall Street Journal* (October 30, 2015), http://www.wsj.com/end-of-life-discussions-will-be-reimbursed-by-medicare-1446240608.

7. Elizabeth B. Lamont and Nicholas A. Christakis, "Prognostic Disclosure to Patients Near the End of Life," *Annals of Internal Medicine* 134 (2001): 1096.

8. Alex Broom et al., "Negotiating Futility, Managing Emotions: Nursing the Transition to Palliative Care," *Qualitative Health Research* 25 (March 2015): 299–309.

9. Ibid.

10. Jerome Groopman and Pamela Hartzband, *Your Medical Mind* (New York: Penguin Books, 2011): 81.

11. Brown, "Denying Death," 54.

12. Ibid., 54.

13. Ibid., 22.

14. Ibid.

15. Atul Gawande, "Letting Go," *The New Yorker* (August 2, 2010): 36–47.

16. Brown, "Denying Death," 32.

17. R. Bhadula, "The Good Physician," *Journal of the American Medical Association* 310, no. 9 (September 4, 2013): 909.

CHAPTER 3

1. Regan Gearhart, "Prehistoric Religion," Indiana University of Pennsylvania (April 25, 2015), http://www.iup.edu/workArea/DownloadAsset.asp?id=193214.

2. Associated Press, "Pope Tells Doctors to Be Wary of 'Extreme Measures,'" *Albuquerque Journal* (March 24, 2002): A11.

3. Katy Butler, *Knocking on Heaven's Door: The Path to a Better Way of Death* (New York: Scribner, 2013), 231.

4. Pope Paul VI, http://www.txcatholic-advance-directives.org/#!terms-of-use/cz5r (accessed December 2, 2015).

5. Centers for Disease Control and Prevention, "Measles—United States, January 4–April 2, 2015" (April 7, 2016), http://www.ced.gov/measles/cases-outbreaks.html.

6. M. C. Shinall, "Fighting for Dear Life: Christians and Aggressive End-of-Life Care," *Perspectives in Biology and Medicine* 57, no. 3 (Summer 2014): 329–40.

7. Christopher Meyers, "Religious Beliefs and Surrogate Medical Decision-making," *Journal of Clinical Ethics* 20, no. 2 (2009): 1.

8. Teneille Brown, "Accommodating Miracles," paper under publication, personal e-mail (August 30, 2015).

9. Wesley J. Smith, *Culture of Death: The Assault on Medical Ethics in America* (San Francisco: Encounter Books, 2000), 131.

10. Ibid., 82.

11. Wesley J. Smith, "Who Decides the Harm in 'Do Not Harm'?" (posted September 29, 2014), http://www.nationalrighttolifenews.org/news/2014/09/who-decides-the-harm-in-do-no-harm/#.VvHDlPkrLcc (accessed November 21, 2014).

12. Catholic Health Association, *Health Progress,* http://www.njha.com/posts/2010/nj-court-has-opportunity-to-influence-compassionate-end-of-life-care/.

13. Shirley Firth, "The End of Life: A Hindu View," *Lancet* 366 (2005): 682–86; Abdulaziz Sachedina, "The End of Life: The Islamic View," *Lancet* 366 (2005): 774–79; Elliot N. Dorff, "The End of Life: Jewish Perspectives," *Lancet* 366 (2005): 862–65; Damien Keown, "The End of Life: The Buddhist View," *Lancet* 366 (2005): 952–55; H. Tristram Engelhardt, Jr., and Ana Smith Iltis, "The End of Life: The Traditional Christian View," *Lancet* 366 (2005): 1045–49; Hazel Markwell, "The End of Life: The Catholic View," *Lancet* 366 (2005): 1132–35; Julian Baggini and Madeleine Pym, "The End of Life: The Humanist View," *Lancet* 366 (2005): 1235–37.

14. Christian Medical and Dental Association, website www.cmda.org (accessed August 31, 2015).

15. Tracy Balboni et al., "Provision of Spiritual Support to Patients with Advanced Cancer by Religious Communities and Associations with Medical Care at the End of Life," *Journal of the American Medical Association* 172, no. 12 (June 24, 2013): 1109.

16. H. Tristram Englehardt, Jr. and Ana Smith Ilitis, "The End of Life: The Traditional Christian View," *Lancet* 3 (2005): 1045–49.

CHAPTER 4

1. K. A. Koch, "Patient Self-Determination Act," *Journal of the Florida Medical Association* 79, no. 4 (April 1992): 240–43.

2. Alfred I. Tauber, quoted in M. Wicclair, "Autonomy Ethics," *Journal of the American Medical Association* 295, no. 20 (May 24/31, 2006): 2416.

3. Abraham Lincoln, "Speech on the Dred Scott Decision" (June 26, 1857), full text, posted on http://teachingamericanhistory.org/library/document/speech-on-the-dred-scott-decision/ (accessed March 23, 2016).

CHAPTER 5

1. Vijay Seshadri, *3 Sections: Poems* (Minneapolis: Graywolf, 2013), http://www.newyorker.com/magazine/2013/11/18/briefly-noted-731 (accessed on March 12, 2013).

2. Katy Butler, *Knocking on Heaven's Door: The Path to a Better Way of Death* (New York: Scribner, 2013), 4.

3. V. S. Periyakoil, E. Neri, A. Fong and H. Kraeme, "Do unto Others: Doctor's Personal End-of-Life Resuscitation Preferences and Their Attitudes Toward Advance Directives," *PLOS ONE* 9, no. 5 (2014): e 98246, doi:10.1371/journal.pone.0098246.

4. Philip A. Pizzo and David M. Walker, "Should We Practice What We Profess? Care Near the End of Life," *New England Journal of Medicine* 372, no. 7 (February 12, 2015): 595–98.

5. Joseph Shapiro, "Why This Wisconsin City Is the Best Place to Die," National Public Radio (first aired November 9, 1009, updated July 14, 2010), accessed online www.npr.org/story/story.php?storyId=120346411.

6. T. E. Quill, R. Arnold and A. L. Back, "Discussing Treatment Preferences with Patients Who Want 'Everything,'" *Annals of Internal Medicine* 151 (2009): 345–49.

7. Thaddeus M. Pope, Pope, "Clinicians May Not Administer Life-Sustaining Treatment Without Consent: Civil, Criminal, and Disciplinary Sanctions," *Journal of Health and Biomedical Law* 9, no. 2 (2013): 213–96. Also http://medicalfutility.blogspot.com/2015/06/no-immunity-for-providers-who-treated.html.

8. Ibid.

9. Butler, *Knocking on Heaven's Door*, 288.

CHAPTER 6

1. Editors of the Encyclopaedia Britannica, "Hippocratic Oath: Ethical Code," *Encyclopaedia Britannica* (November 9, 2014), http://wwwbritannica.som/topic/hippocratic-oath.

2. Gordon Wood, "The Bleeding Founders," *New York Review of Books* (July 10, 2014): 43.

3. Daniel Callahan, *What Kind of Life* (New York: Simon and Schuster, 1991).

4. Helene Starks et al., "Physician Aid-in-Dying," *Ethics in Medicine*, University of Washington School of Medicine (1998, updated 2013), https://depts.washington.edu/bioethx/pad.html.

CHAPTER 7

1. Karen Mizoguchi, "'I'm Going to Live to Be 110 Years Old!' Suzanne Somers, 67, Talks about Life after Breast Cancer and Reveals How She Stays Healthy in a Closer Interview," http://www.dailymail.co.uk/tvshowbiz/article27168689.

2. Angelina Jolie Pitt, "Diary of a Surgery," http://www.nytimes.com/2015/03/24/opinion/angelina-jolie-pitt-diary-of-a-surgery.html.

3. Jerome Groopman and Pamela Hartzband, *Your Medical Mind: How to Decide What Is Right for You* (New York: Penguin Books, 2011), 26.

CHAPTER 8

1. William Osler, "Farewell Dinner Address," Osler Club, London (May 2, 1905).

2. H. Gilbert Welch, Lisa Schwartz and Steve Woloshin, *Overdiagnosed: Making People Sick in the Pursuit of Health* (Boston: Beacon Press, 2011), 15.

3. Mary DeTurris Poust, "Bioethics: What Constitutes 'Extraordinary Means' of Care?" *Our Sunday Visitor* (January 1, 2009), https://www.osv.com/OSVNewsweekly/Story/TabId/2672/ArtMID/13567/ArticleID/13667/Bioethics-What-constitutes-extraordinary-means-of-care.aspx.

4. Atul Gawande, *Being Mortal* (New York: Metropolitan Books, 2014).

5. Ibid., 217–18.

6. Ibid., 220.

7. Diane Meier, quoted by Brett Ryder, *Washington Post* (May 19, 2014), http://patientqualityoflife.org/wp-content/uploads/2014/05/Teaching-doctors-when-to-stop-treatment-The-Washington-Post.pdf (accessed July 24, 2014).

8. William S. Halsted, "The Results of Radical Operations for the Cure of Cancer of the Breast," *Annals of Surgery* (1907): 46.

9. Stephen H. Miles, *The Hippocratic Oath and the Ethics of Medicine* (New York: Oxford University Press, 2004), 30.

10. Maxwell Wintrobe, "The Virtue of Doubt and the Spirit of Inquiry," presidential address to the Association of American Physicians (Atlantic City, May 1965), transcribed by the Association of American Physicians: 78:1. Also quoted in William N. Valentine, "Maxwell Mayer Wintrobe 1901–1986—A Biographical Memoir," National Academy of Sciences (1990), 471.

11. Jerome Groopman and Pamela Hartzband, *Your Medical Mind: How to Decide What Is Right for You* (New York: Penguin, 2011).

12. Ibid., 206.

13. http://www.ascopost.com/ViewNews.aspx?nid=31687.

14. Atul Gawande, "Overkill," *New Yorker* (May 11, 2015): 42.

15. Dennis McCullough, "My Mother, Your Mother: Embracing 'Slow Medicine,' the Compassionate Approach to Caring for Your Aging Loved Ones," reviewed in *Dartmouth Medicine* 32, no. 3 (Spring 2008): 62.

16. H. Gilbert Welch, Lisa Schwartz and Steve Woloshin, *Overdiagnosed* (Boston: Beacon Press, 2011), 62.

17. Deborah Cook and Graeme Rocker, "Dying with Dignity in the Intensive Care Unit," *New England Journal of* Medicine 370, no. 26 (June 26, 2014): 2506–514.

18. ABC News, http://abcnews.go.com/Health/CancerPreventionAndTreatment/steve-jobs-pancreatic-cancer-timeline/story?id=14681812.

CHAPTER 9

1. R. B. Weiss et al., "High Dose Chemotherapy for High Risk Primary Breast Cancer: An On-Site Review of the Bezwoda Study," *Lancet* 355, no. 9208 (March 19, 2000): 999–1003.

2. Katy Butler, *Knocking on Heaven's Door: The Path to a Better Way of Death* (New York: Scribner, 2013).

3. Daren Heyland et al., "The Very Elderly Admitted to ICU: A Quality Finish?" *Critical Care Medicine* 43, no. 7 (July 2015): 1352–60.

4. Tracy Robinson et al., "Patient Oncologist Communication in Advanced Cancer," *Supportive Care in Cancer* 16, no. 9 (January 15, 2008): 1049–57.

5. Gabriel T. Bosslet et al., "An Official ATS/AACN/ACCP/ESICM/SSCM Policy Statement," *American Journal of Respiratory and Critical Care Medicine* 191, no. 11 (June 1, 2015): 1318–30.

6. Susan J. Diem, John D. Lantos and James A. Tulsky, "Cardiopulmonary Resuscitation on Television—Miracles and Misinformation," *New England Journal of Medicine* 334, no. 24 (June 13, 1996): 1578.

7. Jaclyn Portanova et al., "It Isn't like This on Television," *Resuscitation* 96 (August 18, 2015): 148–50.

8. Hideo Yasunaga et al., "Collaborative Effects of Bystander-initiated Cardiopulmonary Resuscitation and Prehospital Advanced Cardiac Life Support by Physicians on Survival of Out-of-Hospital Cardiac Arrest: A Nationwide Population-Based Observational Study," *Critical Care* 14 (November 4, 2010): R199, http://ccforum.com/content/14/6/R199.

9. Paul A. Manner, "Practicing Defensive Medicine—Not Good for Patients or Physicians," *American Association of Orthopaedic Surgeons, AAOS Now* (January–February 2007).

10. Tom Baker, *The Myth of Medical Malpractice* (Chicago: University of Chicago Press, 2007).

11. Emily Carrier et al., "Physicians' Fears of Malpractice Are Not Assuaged by Tort Reforms," *Health Affairs* 29 (September 2010): 1585–92.

12. Daniel A. Waxman et al., "The Effect of Malpractice Reform on Emergency Medical Department Care," *New England Journal of Medicine* 371 (October 16, 2014): 1518–25.

13. Arnold S. Relman, "The New Medical Industrial Complex," *New England Journal of Medicine* 303, no. 17 (October 23, 1980): 963–70.

14. Joseph A. Ladapo, Saul Blecker and Pamela S. Douglas, "Physician Decision-making and Trends in the Use of Cardiac Stress Testing in the United States: An Analysis of Repeated Cross-Sectional Data," *Annals of Internal Medicine* 161, no. 7 (October 7, 2014): 482–90.

15. Teneille Brown, "Denying Death," *Arizona Law Review* 56, no. 4 (2015): 127.

16. Anna Wilde Matthews and Lisa Schwartz, "Medicare Paid One Doctor More than $20 Million in 2012," *Wall Street Journal* (April 9, 2014).

17. Medicare, "Medicare Coverage of Kidney Dialysis and Kidney Transplants," https://www.medicare.govv/Pubs/pdf/10128.pdf.

18. Sandeep Jauhar, *Doctored* (New York: Farrar, Straus and Giroux, 2015), 97.

19. Thomas J. Smith and Bruce E. Hillner, "Bending the Cost Curve in Cancer Care," *New England Journal of Medicine* 364, no. 21 (May 26, 2011): 2060.

20. American Society of Clinical Oncology, http://oncology.jamanetwork.com/article.aspx?articleid=2398177.

21. L. N. Newcomer et al., "Changing Physician Incentives for Affordable, Quality Cancer Care: Results of an Episode Payment Model," *Journal of Oncology Practice* 10, no. 5 (September 1, 2014): 322–26. doi:10.1200/*Journal of Oncology Practice*.2014.001488.

22. Alan Bavley, *Kansas City Star* (posted January 27, 2009), http://www.kansascity.com/story/1293202-p2.html (accessed July 24, 2014).

23. Office of the Inspector General, Department of Health and Human Services, "Improper Payments for Evaluation and Management Services Cost Medicare Billions in 2010," http://www.oig.hhs/gov/oei/reports/oei-04-10-0081.pdf.

24. Atul Gawande, "The Cost Conundrum," *New Yorker* (June 1, 2009).

25. Patrick Radden Keefe, "The Empire Edge," *New Yorker* (October 13, 2014): 76.

26. G. E. Kaebnick, "Too Sick," *Hastings Center Report* 42, no. 2 (2012), doi: 10.1002/hast.55.

27. James Surowieki, "Bitter Pill," *New Yorker* (May 2, 2011): 25.

28. Teneille Brown, "Denying Death," *Arizona Law Review* 56, no. 4:1 (2015): 53.

29. Ibid.

30. http://www.medscape.com/viewarticle/853541 (accessed March 24, 2016).

31. Jed S. Rakoff, "Justice Deferred Is Justice Denied," *New York Review of Books* (February 19, 2015): 10.

32. Christina A. Sarich, "Big Pharma Spends $65.4 Million on Lobbying in Q1 of 2014," *Nation of Change* (May 17, 2014), http://www.nationofchange.org/big-pharma-spends-big-lobbying-q1-2014-1400337153 (accessed May 19, 2014).

33. Ben Goldacre, *Bad Pharma: How Drug Companies Mislead Doctors and Harm Patients* (New York: Faber and Faber, Inc., 2012).

34. National Cancer Institute, "FDA Approval for Bevacizumab," http.//www.cancer.gov/about-cancer/treatment/drugs/fda-bevacizumab#Anchor-Metastati-43353.

35. Joe Nocera, "Why Doesn't No Mean No?" *New York Times* (November 20, 2011): A29.

36. Katy Butler, *Knocking on Heaven's Door: The Path to a Better way of Death* (New York: Scribner, 2013), 171.

37. Pierluigi Tricoci, quoted in Butler, *Knocking on Heaven's Door*, 178.

38. Lara Goitein, review of Kenneth M. Ludmerer's *Let Me Heal: The Opportunity to Preserve Excellence in American Medicine* (New York: Oxford University Press, 2014) in *New York Review of Books* (June 5, 2015): 60.

39. Ibid.

40. Daniel Callahan, *The Research Imperative: What Price Better Health?* (Oakland: University of California Press, 2003).

41. Centers for Disease Control and Prevention, "Leading Causes of Death 1900–1998," http://www.cdc.gov/nchs/data/dvs/lead1900_98.pdf, and "FastStats: Leading Causes of Death," http://www.cdc.gov/nchs/fastats/leading-causes-of-death.htm.

42. Daniel Callahan, *False Hopes* (New Brunswick: Rutgers University Press, 1999), 241.

43. Vincent T. DeVita, Jr., *The Death of Cancer* (New York: Sarah Crichton Books, Farrar, Straus and Giroux, 2015).

44. Justin E. Bekelman, Yan Li and Cary P. Gross, "Impact of Financial Conflicts of Interest in Biomedical Research," *Journal of the American Medical Association* 289, no. 4 (January 20, 2003): 454–65.

45. David Kent, "Scientific Integrity," *Journal of the American Medical Association* 295, no. 20 (May 2006): 2418.

46. Yale Cancer Center and Smilow Cancer Hospital, "Breakthroughs: The Year in Review" (2013): 16, https://medicine,yale.edu/cancer/news/YCC_2013Breakthroughs_020514_177444_12062.pdf.

47. Peter Whoriskey, "Doubts about Johns Hopkins Research Have Gone Unanswered, Scientist Says," *Washington Post* (March 11, 2013), https://www.washingtonpost.com/business/economy/doubts-about- johns-hopkins-research-have-gone- unanswered-scientist- says/2013/03/11/52822cba-7c84- 11e2-82e8-61a46c2cde3d_story.html.

48. Duff Wilson and David Heath, "The Blood Cancer Experiment: Patients Never Knew the Full Danger of Trials They Staked Their Lives On," *Seattle Times* (2001), http://old.seattletimes.com/uninformed_consent/bloodcancer/story1.html.

49. University of Pennsylvania, "US Settles Case of Gene Therapy Study that Ended with Teen's Death," *University of Pennsylvania Almanac* 51, no. 21 (February 15, 2015), http://www.upenn.edu/almanac/volumes/v51/n21/gts.html.

50. Carl Elliott, "The University of Minnesota's Medical Research Mess," *New York Times* (May 26, 2015): A19.

CHAPTER 10

1. Thaddeus Pope, http://medicalfutility.blogspot.com/2014/09/overemphasis-on-errors-of-unwanted.html.

2. Tamar Lewin, "Nancy Cruzan Dies, Outlived by a Debate over the Right to Die," *New York Times* (December 27, 1990), http.//www.nytimes.com/1990/12/27/us/nancy-cruzan-dies-outlived-by-a-debate-over-the-right-to-die.html.

3. Jerome Groopman and Pamela Hartzband, *Your Medical Mind: How to Decide What Is Right for You* (New York: Penguin, 2011), 183.

4. Daniel Callahan, "Death and the Research Imperative," *New England Journal of Medicine* 342, no. 9 (March 2, 2000): 654–56.

5. Tracy A. Balboni et al., "Provision of Spiritual Support to Patients with Advanced Cancer by Religious Communities and Associations with Medical Care at the End of Life," *Journal of the American Medical Association Internal Medicine* 173, no. 12 (June 24, 2013): 1109–17.

CHAPTER 11

1. Gabriel T. Bosslet, et al., "An Official ATS/AACN/ACCP/ESICM/SCCM Policy Statement: Responding to Requests for Potentially Inappropriate Treatments in Intensive Care Units," *American Journal of Respiratory and Critical Care Medicine* 191, no. 11 (June 1, 2015): 1318–30.

2. Council on Ethical and Judicial Affairs, American Medical Association, *Journal of American Medical Association* 281, no. 10 (March 10, 1999): 937.

3. Institute of Medicine, "Dying in America," September 2014. Accessed February 20, 2015, http://www.nationalacademies.org/hmd/~/media/Files/Report%20Files/2014/EOL/Key%20Findings%20and%20Recommendations.pdf.

4. Wesley J. Smith, *Culture of Death: The Assault on Medical Ethics in America* (San Francisco: Encounter Books, 2000), 85.

5. Kathryn Tucker, http://www.disabilityrightslegalcenter@lls.edu (accessed May 15, 2014).

CHAPTER 12

1. Stephen Brill, "Bitter Pill: Why Medical Bills Are Killing Us," *Time* (March 4, 2013): 18–54.

2. Peggy Orenstein, "Our Feel Good War on Breast Cancer," *New York Times* (April 25, 2013), http://www.nytimes.com/2013/04/28/magazine/our-feel-good-war-on-breast-cancer.html (accessed June 15, 2013).

3. Institute of Medicine, "Unequal Treatment: Confronting Racial and Ethnic Disparities in Health Care" (2002), http://www.nationalacademies.org/hmd/Reports/2002/Unequal-Treatment-Confronting-Racial-and-Ethnic-Disparities-in-Health-Care.aspx.

4. R. Wyatt and D. R. Williams, "Racial Bias in Health Care and Health," *Journal of the American Medical Association* 314, no. 6 (August 11, 2015): 555.

5. Robert D. Truog, "Medical Futility," *Georgia State University Law Review* (2009): 985.

6. Preethy Nayar, "Disparities in End of Life Care for Elderly Lung Cancer Patients," *Journal of Community Health* 29 (2014): 1012.

7. Amresh Hanchate et al., "Racial and Ethnic Differences in End-of-Life Costs: Why Do Minorities Cost More Than Whites?" *Archives of Internal Medicine* 169, no. 5 (2009): 493–501.

8. Bernie S. Siegel, *Love, Medicine and Miracles* (London: Arrow Books, 1988).

9. American Society of Clinical Oncology, *Journal of Clinical Oncology* 61 (2015): 6706.

10. Julian Barnes, "'For Sorrow There Is No Remedy,'" *New York Review of Books* 58, no. 6 (April 7, 2011).

11. Teneille Brown, "Accommodating Miracles," paper under publication, personal email (accessed August 30, 2015).

12. Butler, *Knocking on Heaven's Door*, 195.

13. Bill Hutchinson, "Christopher Reeve Dies, 52, in 2004," *New York Daily News* (October 11, 2004), www.nydailynews.com/entertainment/christopher-reeve-dies-52-2004-article1.575826.

14. Katie Thomas, "In Race for Medicare Dollars, Nursing Home Care May Lag," *New York Times* (April 14, 2015): B1.

15. Butler, *Knocking on Heaven's Door*, 31.

CHAPTER 13

1. Teneille Brown, "Denying Death," *Arizona Law Review* 56, no. 4 (2015): 1.

2. Laura Tenner and Paul R. Helft, "In Search of Value in Cancer Care: What Resources Are Available to Practicing Oncologists?" *The Oncology Journal* 29, no. 10 (October 2015): 783–85.

3. Ibid.

4. Atul Gawande, "The Cost Conundrum," *New Yorker* (June 1, 2009): 36–44.

5. Brown, "Denying Death," 55.

6. Kimberly Leonard, "Medicare Rule Revisits 'Death Panel' Issue," *US News and World Report* (July 9, 2015), http://www.usnews.com/news/articles/2015/07/09/medicare-rule-revisits-death-panel-issue.html.

7. Brown, "Accommodating Miracles," paper under publication, personal e-mail (accessed August 30, 2015).

8. Kristin M. Kostick and Jennifer Blumenthal-Barby, "The Device Kept Him Alive, but Was the Pain and Suffering Worth It?" *Washington Post* (August 3, 2015), http://www.washingtonpost.com/health-science.html.

9. Charles D. Blanke and Erik K. Fromme, "Chemotherapy Near the End of Life: First—and Third and Fourth (Line)—Do No Harm," *JAMA Oncology* 1, no. 6 (September 2015): 785–86.

10. *Merriam Webster Dictionary* online, http://www.merriam-webster.com/dictionary/palliative (accessed March 24, 2016).

11. Sarah Elizabeth Harrington and Thomas J. Smith, "The Role of Chemotherapy at the End of Life: When Is Enough, Enough?" *Journal of the American Medical Association* 229, no. 22 (June 11, 2008): 2667–78.

12. Isablelle Baszanger, "One More Chemo or One Too Many? Defining the Limits of Treatment and Innovation in Medical Oncology," *Social Science and Medicine* 75, no. 5 (September 2012): 864–72.

13. Sean Cole, Joseph Gallo and Ken Murray, "The Bitter End" (January 15, 2013), http://www.radiolab.org/story/262588-bitter-end/ (accessed February 26, 2014).

14. Katy Butler, *Knocking on Heaven's Door*, 4.

15. Jennifer S. Temel et al., "Early Palliative Care for Patients with Metastatic Non–Small-Cell Lung Cancer," *New England Journal of Medicine* 363, no. 8 (August 19, 2010): 733–42.

16. Denys Cope, *Dying: A Natural Passage* (Santa Fe: Three Whales Publishing, 2008), 4.

17. Holly G. Prigerson and Selby C. Jacobs, "Caring for Bereaved Patients 'All the Doctors Just Suddenly Go'," *Journal of the American Medical Association* 286, no. 11 (September 19, 2001): 1369–76.

18. Catholics United for the Faith, "The Principle of Double Effect" (1997), http://www.cuf.org/FileDownloads/doubleeffect.pdf.

19. Antonia Blumberg, "Nearly 70 percent of Americans Support Euthanasia, but Opinions Vary by Religiosity," *Huffington Post* (June 19, 2014), http://www.huffingtonpost.com/2014/06/19/americans-support-euthanasia_n_5510949.html (accessed July 20, 2014).

20. David Orentlicher, Thaddeus M. Pope and Ben A. Rich, "The Changing Legal Climate for Physician Aid in Dying," *Journal of the American Medical Association* 311, no. 19 (May 21, 2014): 1961–62.

21. Elizabeth Trice Loggers et al., "Implementing a Death with Dignity Program at a Comprehensive Cancer Center," *New England Journal of Medicine* 368, no. 15 (April 11, 2013): 1417–24.

22. Council of Catholic Bishops, http://wwwmigrate.usccb.org/issues-and-action/human-life-and-dignity/assisted-suicide/to-live-each-day/upload/to-live-each-day-with-dignity-hyperlinked.pdf (accessed August 12, 2013).

23. Maria L. LaGagna, "Death with Dignity Act in Oregon: A Preview of What California Might Expect," *Los Angeles Times* (October 8, 2015), http://www.latimes.com/national/a-n:-oregon-assisted-suicide-2015/10/08-story.html.

24. Ibid.

25. Steven H. Miles, *The Hippocratic Oath and the Ethics of Medicine* (New York: Oxford University Press, 2004), 68.

26. Tony Delamothe, Rosamund Snow and Fiona Godlee, "Why the Assisted Dying Bill should become law in England and Wales," *British Medical Journal* 349 (published July 2, 2014), http://dx.doi.org/10.1136/bmj.g4349.

27. Orentlicher et al., "The Changing Legal Climate," 1961–62.

28. Richard Horton, "Fibbing for God," *Lancet* 386, no. 9997 (September 5, 2015): 940.

29. Ibid.

30. Zanny Minton-Beddoes, "Doctor-Assisted Dying: The Right to Die," *Economist* (June 27, 2015): 21, http://www.economist.com/news/leaders/21656182-doctors-should-be-allowed-help-suffering-and-terminally-ill-die-when-they-choose (accessed July 15, 2015).

31. Thomas Beauchamp and James Childers, *Principles of Biomedical Ethics*, 5th ed. (New York: Oxford University Press, 2001), 39.

32. Reinhold Niebuhr, http://www.aahistory.com/prayer.html.

Bibliography

ABC News. http://abcnews.go.com/Health/CancerPreventionAndTreatment/steve-jobs-pancreatic-cancer-timeline/story?id=14681812.

American Society of Clinical Oncology. *Journal of Clinical Oncology* 61 (2015).

American Society of Clinical Oncology. http://oncology.jamanetwork.com/article.aspx?articleid=2398177.

Armour, Stephanie. "End-of-Life Discussions Will Be Reimbursed by Medicare." *Wall Street Journal* (October 30, 2015). http://www.wsj.com/end-of-life-discussions-will-be-reimbursed-by-medicare-1446240608.

Baggini, Julian and Madeleine Pym. "The End of Life: The Humanist View." *Lancet* 366 (2005): 9486–515.

Balboni, Tracy A., et al. "Provision of Spiritual Support to Patients with Advanced Cancer by Religious Communities and Associations with Medical Care at the End of Life." *Journal of the American Medical Association Internal Medicine* 173, no. 12 (June 24, 2013).

Baker, Tom. 2007. *The Myth of Medical Malpractice.* 1st ed. Chicago: University of Chicago Press.

Barnes, Julian. "'For Sorrow There Is No Remedy.'" *New York Review of Books* 58, no. 6 (April 7, 2011).

Baszanger, Isabelle. "One More Chemo or One Too Many? Defining the Limits of Treatment and Innovation in Medical Oncology." *Social Science and Medicine* 75, no. 5 (September 2, 2012).

Bavley, Alan. *Kansas City Star* (posted January 27, 2009). http://www.kansascity.com/story/1293202-p2.html. Accessed June 30, 2009.

Beauchamp, Thomas and James Childers. 2001. *Principles of Biomedical Ethics*. 5th ed. New York: Oxford University Press.

Bekelman, Justin E., Yan Li and Cary P. Gross. "Impact of Financial Conflicts of Interest in Biomedical Research." *Journal of the American Medical Association* 289, no. 4 (January 20, 2003).

Bhadula, R. "The Good Physician." *Journal of the American Medical Association* 310, no. 9 (September 4, 2013).

Blanke, Charles D., and Erik K. Fromme. "Chemotherapy near the End of Life: First— and Third and Fourth (Line)—Do No Harm." *JAMA Oncology* 1, no. 6 (September 2015).

Blumberg, Antonia. "Nearly 70 percent of Americans Support Euthanasia, but Opinions Vary by Religiosity." *Huffington Post* (June 19, 2014). http://www.huffingtonpost.com/2014/06/19/americans-support-euthanasia_n_5510949.html. Accessed July 20, 2014.

Bosslet, Gabriel T., et al. "An Official ATS/AACN/ACCP/ESICM/SCCM Policy Statement: Responding to Requests for Potentially Inappropriate Treatments in Intensive Care Units." *American Journal of Respiratory and Critical Care Medicine* 191, no. 11 (June 1, 2015).

Brill, Stephen. "Bitter Pill: Why Medical Bills Are Killing Us." *Time* (March 4, 2013).

Broom, Alex, et al. "Negotiating Futility, Managing Emotions: Nursing the Transition to Palliative Care." *Qualitative Health Research* 25 (March 2015).

Brown, Teneille. "Accommodating Miracles," paper under publication, personal e-mail. Accessed August 30, 2015.

———. "Denying Death." *Arizona Law Review* 56, no. 4 (2015).

Butler, Katy. 2013. *Knocking on Heaven's Door: The Path to a Better Way of Death*. New York: Scribner.

Callahan, Daniel. 1991. *What Kind of Life*. New York: Simon and Schuster.

———. 1999. *False Hopes*. New Brunswick: Rutgers University Press.

———. "Death and the Research Imperative." *New England Journal of Medicine* 342, no. 9 (March 2, 2000).

———. 2003. *The Research Imperative: What Price Better Health?* Oakland: University of California Press.

Carrier, Emily et al. "Physicians' Fears of Malpractice Are Not Assuaged by Tort Reforms." *Health Affairs* 29 (September 2010).

Catholic Health Association. *Health Progress*. http://www.njha.com/posts/2010/nj-court-has-opportunity-to-influence-compassionate-end-of-life-care/.

Catholics United for the Faith. "The Principle of Double Effect" (1997). http://www.cuf.org/FileDownloads/doubleeffect.pdf.

Centers for Disease Control and Prevention. "Leading Causes of Death 1900–1998," http://www.cdc.gov/nchs/data/dvs/lead1900_98.pdf, and "FastStats: Leading Causes of Death," http://www.cdc.gov/nchs/fastats/leading-causes-of-death.htm.

Centers for Disease Control and Prevention. "Measles—United States, January 4–April 2, 2015" (April 7, 2016). http.//www.ced.gov/measles/cases-outbreaks.html.

Centers for Disease Control and Prevention. "U.S. Public Health Service Syphilis Study at Tuskegee" (February 19, 2016). http://www.cdc.gov/tuskegee/timline.html.

Christian Medical and Dental Association. http://www.cmda.org. Accessed August 31, 2015.

Cole, Sean, Joseph Gallo and Ken Murray. "The Bitter End" (January 15, 2013). http://www.radiolab.org/story/262588-bitter-end/. Accessed February 26, 2014.

Cook, Deborah and Graeme Rocker. "Dying with Dignity in the Intensive Care Unit." *New England Journal of* Medicine 370, no. 26 (June 26, 2014).

Cope, Denys. 2008. *Dying: A Natural Passage.* Santa Fe: Three Whales Publishing.

Council of Catholic Bishops. http://wwwmigrate.usccb.org/issues-and-action/human-life-and-dignity/assisted-suicide/to-live-each-day/upload/to-live-each-day-with-dignity-hyperlinked.pdf.

Council on Ethical and Judicial Affairs, American Medical Association. *Journal of the American Medical Association* 281, no. 10 (March 10, 1999).

DeVita, Vincent T., Jr. 2015. *The Death of Cancer.* New York: Sarah Crichton Books, Farrar, Straus and Giroux.

Delamothe, Tony, Rosamund Snow and Fiona Godlee. "Why the Assisted Dying Bill Should Become Law in England and Wales." *British Medical Journal* 349 (published July 2, 1014). http://dx.doi.org/10.1136/bmj.g4349.

Diem, Suwsan J., John D. Lantos and James A. Tulsky. "Cardiopulmonary Resuscitation on Television—Miracles and Misinformation." *New England Journal of Medicine* 334, no. 24 (June 13, 1996).

Dorff, Elliott N. "The End of Life: Jewish Perspectives." *Lancet* 366 (2005).

Editors of the Encyclopaedia Britannica. "Hippocratic Oath: Ethical Code." *Encyclopaedia Britannica* (November 9, 2014). http://wwwbritannica.som/topic/hippocratic-oath.

Elliott, Carl. "The University of Minnesota's Medical Research Mess." *New York Times* (May 26, 2015).

Englehardt, H. Tristram, Jr. and Ana Smith Ilitis. "The End of Life: The Traditional Christian View." *Lancet* 366 (2005).

Firth, Shirley. "The End of Life: A Hindu View." *Lancet* 366 (2005).

Furrow, Barry et al. 2013. *Bioethics: Healthcare Law and Ethics*, 7th ed. St. Paul: West Academic Publishing.

Gawande, Atul. "The Cost Conundrum." *New Yorker* (June 1, 2009).

———. "Letting Go." *New Yorker* (August 2, 2010).

———. 2014. *Being Mortal*. New York: Metropolitan Books.

———. "Overkill." *New Yorker* (May 11, 2015).

Gearhart, Regan. "Prehistoric Religion." Indiana University of Pennsylvania (April 25, 2015). http.://www.iup.edu/workArea/DownloadAsset.asp?id=193214.

Goitein, Lara. Review of Kenneth M. Ludmerer's *Let Me Heal: The Opportunity to Preserve Excellence in American Medicine* (New York: Oxford University Press, 2014) in *New York Review of Books* (June 5, 2015).

Goldacre, Ben. 2012. *Bad Pharma: How Drug Companies Mislead Doctors and Harm Patients*. New York: Faber and Faber, Inc.

Groopman, Jerome and Pamela Hartzband. 2011. *Your Medical Mind: How to Decide What Is Right for You*. New York: Penguin Books.

Halifax, Joan. "Compassion and the True Meaning of Empathy." TED (posted September 2011). https://www.ted.com/talks/joan_halifax/transcript?language=en.

Halsted, William S. "The Results of Radical Operations for the Cure of Cancer of the Breast." *Annals of Surgery* 46, no. 1 (July 1907): 1–19.

Hanchate, Amresh et al. "Racial and Ethnic Differences in End-of-Life Costs: Why Do Minorities Cost More Than Whites?" *Archives of Internal Medicine* 169, no. 5 (2009).

Hansen, Terri. "Unethical Medical Experiments Still a Possibility." Indian Country Today Media Network.com (March 10, 2011). http://www.indiancountrytoday-medianetwork.com/2011/03/10/unethical-medical-experiments-still-a-possibility.html.

Harrintgon, Sarah Elizabeth and Thomas J. Smith. "The Role of Chemotherapy at the End of Life: When is Enough, Enough?" *Journal of the American Medical Association* 229, no. 22 (June 11, 2008).

Heyland, Daren et al. "The Very Elderly Admitted to ICU: A Quality Finish?" *Critical Care Medicine* 43, no. 7 (July 2015).

Horton, Richard. "Fibbing for God." *Lancet* 386, no. 9997 (September 5, 2015).

Hutchinson, Bill. "Christopher Reeve Dies, 52, in 2004." *New York Daily News* (October 11, 2004), www.nydailynews.com/entertainment/christopher-reeve-dies-52-2004-article1.575826.

Institute of Medicine. "Dying in America." September 2014. http://www. nationalacademies.org/hmd/~/media/Files/Report%20Files/2014/EOL/Key%20 Findings%20and%20Recommendations.pdf. Accessed February 20, 2015.

Institute of Medicine. 2002. "Unequal Treatment: Confronting Racial and Ethnic Disparities in Health Care." http://www.nationalacademies.org/hmd/Reports/2002/ Unequal-Treatment-Confronting-Racial-and-Ethnic-Disparities-in-Health-Care. aspx.

Jauhar, Sandeep. 2015. *Doctored*. New York: Farrar, Straus and Giroux.

Kaebnick, G. E. "Too Sick." *Hastings Center Report* 42, no. 2 (2012). doi: 10.1002/ hast.55.

Keefe, Patrick Radden. "The Empire Edge." *New Yorker* (October 13, 2014).

Kent, David. "Scientific Integrity." *Journal of the American Medical Association* 295, no. 20 (May 2006).

Keown, Damien. "The End of Life: The Buddhist View." *Lancet* 366 (2005).

Koch, K. A. "Patient Self-Determination Act." *Journal of the Florida Medical Association* 79, no. 4 (April 1992): 240–43.

Koh, H. K. "The Arc of Health Literacy." *Journal of the American Medical Association* 314, no. 12 (September 22/29, 2015).

Kostick, Kristin M., and Jennifer Blumenthal-Barby. "The Device Kept Him Alive, but Was the Pain and Suffering Worth It?" *Washington Post* (August 3, 2015). http:// www.washingtonpost.com/health-science.html.

Kübler-Ross, Elisabeth. 1969. *On Death and Dying*. New York: MacMillan.

Ladapo, Joseph A., Saul Blecker and Pamela S. Douglas. "Physician Decision-making and Trends in the Use of Cardiac Stress Testing in the United States: An Analysis of Repeated Cross-Sectional Data." *Annals of Internal Medicine* 161, no. 7 (October 7, 2014).

LaGagna, Maria L. "Death with Dignity Act in Oregon: A Preview of What California Might Expect." *Los Angeles Times* (October 8, 2015). http://www.latimes.com/ national/a-n:-oregon-assisted-suicide-2015/10/08-story.html.

Lamont, Elizabeth B., and Nicholas A. Christakis. "Prognostic Disclosure to Patients near the End of Life." *Annals of Internal Medicine* 134 (2001).

Leonard, Kimberly. "Medicare Rule Revisits 'Death Panel' Issue." *US News and World Report* (July 9, 2015). http://www.usnews.com/news/articles/2015/07/09/medicare-rule-revisits-death-panel-issue.html.

Lewin, Tamar. "Nancy Cruzan Dies, Outlived by a Debate over the Right to Die." *New York Times* (December 27, 1990). http.//www.nytimes.com/1990/12/27/us/nancy-cruzan-dies-outlived-by-a-debate-over-the-right-to-die.html.

Lincoln, Abraham. "Speech on the Dred Scott Decision" (June 26, 1857). Full text posted on http://teachingamericanhistory.org/library/document/speech-on-the-dred-scott-decision/.

Logggers, Elizabeth Trice et al. "Implementing a Death with Dignity Program at a Comprehensive Cancer Center." *New England Journal of Medicine* 368, no. 15 (April 11, 2013).

Mangan, Dan. "Medical Bills Are the Biggest Cause of US Bankruptcy: Study." CNBC (June 25, 2013). http://www.cnbc.com/id/100840148.html.

Manner, Paul A. "Practicing Defensive Medicine—Not Good for Patients or Physicians." American Association of Orthopaedic Surgeons, *AAOS Now* (January–February 2007).

Markwell, Hazel. "The End of Life: The Catholic View." *Lancet* 366 (2005).

Matthews, Anna Wile and Lisa Schwartz. "Medicare Paid One Doctor More than $20 Million in 2012." *Wall Street Journal* (April 9, 2014).

McCullough, Dennis. "My Mother, Your Mother: Embracing 'Slow Medicine,' the Compassionate Approach to Caring for Your Aging Loved Ones." Reviewed in *Dartmouth Medicine* 32, no. 3 (Spring 2008).

Medicare. "Medicare Coverage of Kidney Dialysis and Kidney Transplants." https://www.medicare.govv/Pubs/pdf/10128.pdf.

Merriam Webster Dictionary online. http://www.merriam-webster.com/dictionary/palliative. Accessed March 24, 2016.

Meyers, Christopher. "Religious Beliefs and Surrogate Medical Decision-making." *Journal of Clinical Ethics* 20, no. 2 (2009).

Miles, Steven H. 2004. *The Hippocratic Oath and the Ethics of Medicine*. New York: Oxford University Press.

Minton-Beddoes, Zanny. "Doctor-Assisted Dying: The Right to Die." *Economist* (June 27, 2015): 21. Online: http://www.economist.com/news/leaders/21656182-doctors-should-be-allowed-help-suffering-and-terminally-ill-die-when-they-choose.

Mizoguchi, Karen. "'I'm Going to Live to Be 110 Years Old!' Suzanne Somers, 67, Talks about Life after Breast Cancer and Reveals How She Stays Healthy in a Closer Interview." http://www.dailymail.co.uk/tvshowbiz/article27168689.

National Cancer Institute. "FDA Approval for Bevacizumab." http://www.cancer.gov/about-cancer/treatment/drugs/fda-bevacizumab#Anchor-Metastati-43353.

National Cancer Institute. "Milestone (1971): National Cancer Act of 1971." https://dtp.cancer.gov/timeline/flash/milestone/M4_Nixon.htm.

Nayar, Preethy. "Disparities in End of Life Care for Elderly Lung Cancer Patients." *Journal of Community Health* 29 (2014).

Newcomer, Lee N., Bruce Gould, Ray D. Page, Sheila A. Donelan and Monica Perkins. "Changing Physician Incentives for Affordable, Quality Cancer Care, Results of an Episode Payment Model." *Journal of Oncology Practice* 10, no. 5 (September 2014): 322–26.

Niebuhr, Reinhold. http://www.aahistory.com/prayer.html.

Nocera, Joe. "Why Doesn't No Mean No?" *New York Times* (November 20, 2011).

Nuland, Sherwin. 1993. *How We Die: Reflections on Life's Final Chapter*. New York: Vintage Books.

Office of the Inspector General, Department of Health and Human Services. "Improper Payments for Evaluation and Management Services Cost Medicare Billions in 2010." http://www.oig.hhs/gov/oei/reports/oei-04-10-0081.pdf.

Orenstein, Peggy. "Our Feel Good War on Breast Cancer." *New York Times* (April 25, 2013). http://www.nytimes.com/2013/04/28/magazine/our-feel-good-war-on-breast-cancer.html. Accessed June 15, 2013.

Orentlicher, David, Thaddeus M. Pope and Ben A. Rich. "The Changing Legal Climate for Physician Aid in Dying." *Journal of the American Medical Association* 311, no. 19 (May 21, 2014).

Osler, William. "Farewell Dinner Address." Osler Club, London (May 2, 1905).

Periyakoil, V. S., E. Neri, A. Fong and H. Kraeme. "Do unto Others: Doctor's Personal End-of-Life Resuscitation Preferences and Their Attitudes toward Advance Directives." *PLos One* 9, no. 5 (2014): e 98246. doi:10.1371/journal.pone.0098246.

Pitt, Angelina Jolie. "Diary of a Surgery." http://www.nytimes.com/2015/03/24/opinion/angelina-jolie-pitt-diary-of-a-surgery.html.

Pizzo, Philip A., and David M. Walker. "Should We Practice What We Profess? Care Near the End of Life." *New England Journal of Medicine* 372, no. 7 (February 12, 2015).

Pope, Thaddeus M. "Clinicians May Not Administer Life-Sustaining Treatment without Consent: Civil, Criminal, and Disciplinary Sanctions." *Journal of Health and Biomedical Law* 9, no. 2 (2013): 213–96. Also http://medicalfutility.blogspot.com/2015/06/no-immunity-for-providers-who-treated.html.

———. http://medicalfutility.blogspot.com/2014/09/overemphasis-on-errors-of-unwanted.html.

Portanova, Jaclyn et al. "It Isn't Like This on Television." *Resuscitation* 96 (August 18, 2015).

Poust, Mary DeTurris. "Bioethics: What Constitutes 'Extraordinary Means' of Care?" *Our Sunday Visitor* (January 1, 2009). https://www.osv.com/OSVNewsweekly/Story/TabId/2672/ArtMID/13567/ArticleID/13667/Bioethics-What-constitutes-extraordinary-means-of-care.aspx.

Prigerson, Holly G., and Selby C. Jacobs. "Caring for Bereaved Patients 'All the Doctors Just Suddenly Go.'" *Journal of the American Medical Association* 286, no. 11 (September 19, 2001).

Quill, T. E., R. Arnold and A. L. Back. "Discussing Treatment Preferences with Patients Who Want 'Everything.'" *Annals of Internal Medicine* 151 (2009).

Rakoff, Jed S. "Justice Deferred Is Justice Denied." *New York Review of Books* (February 19, 2015).

Relman, Arnold S. "The New Medical Industrial Complex." *New England Journal of Medicine* 303, no. 17 (October 23, 1980).

Robinson, Tracy et al. "Patient Oncologist Communication in Advanced Cancer." *Supportive Care in Cancer* 16, no. 9 (January 15, 2008): 1049–57.

Ryder, Brett. *Washington Post* (May 19, 2014). http://patientqualityoflife.org/wp-content/uploads/2014/05/Teaching-doctors-when-to-stop-treatment-The-Washington-Post.pdf. Accessed July 24, 2014.

Sachedina, Abdulaziz. "The End of Life: The Islamic View." *Lancet* 366 (2005).

Sacred Texts. "The Mustard Seed." http://www.sacredtexts.com/bud/btg/btg85.htm.

Sarich, Christina A. "Big Pharma Spends $65.4 Million on Lobbying in Q1 of 2014." *Nation of Change* (May 17, 2014). http://www.nationofchange.org/big-pharma-spends-big-lobbying-q1-2014-1400337153. Accessed May 19, 2014.

Seshadri, Vijay. 2013. *3 Sections: Poems.* Minneapolis: Graywolf.

Shapiro, Joseph. "Why this Wisconsin City Is the Best Place to Die." National Public Radio (first aired November 16, 2009, updated July 14, 2010). Accessed online www.npr.org/story/story.php?storyId=120346411.

Shinall, M. C. "Fighting for Dear Life: Christians and Aggressive End-of-Life Care." *Perspectives in Biology and Medicine* 57, no. 3 (Summer 2014).

Siegel, Bernie S. 1988. *Love, Medicine and Miracles.* London: Arrow Books.

Smith, Thomas J., and Bruce E. Hillner. "Bending the Cost Curve in Cancer Care." *New England Journal of Medicine* 364, no. 21 (May 26, 2011).

Smith, Wesley J. 2000. *Culture of Death: The Assault on Medical Ethics in America.* San Francisco: Encounter Books.

———. "Futile Care Theory: Bioethicists Should Stop Pretending They Are Doing Patients a Favor" (posted May 30, 2010). http://www.firstthings.com/blogs/

firstthoughts/2010/05/futile-care-theory-bioethicists-should-stop-pretending-they-are-doing-patients-a-favor. Accessed January 10, 2015.

———. "Who Decides the Harm in 'Do Not Harm'?" (posted September 29, 2014). http://www.nationalrighttolifenews.org/news/2014/09/who-decides-the-harm-in-do-no-harm/#.VvHDlPkrLcc. Accessed November 21, 2014.

———. "Medicare and Medical Futility." *The Weekly Standard* 21, no. 10 (November 16, 2015).

Starks, Helene et al. "Physician Aid-in-Dying." *Ethics in Medicine*, University of Washington School of Medicine (1998, updated 2013). https://depts.washington.edu/bioethx/pad.html.

Surowieki, James. "Bitter Pill." *New Yorker* (May 2, 2011).

Tenner, Laura and Paul R. Helft. "In Search of Value in Cancer Care: What Resources Are Available to Practicing Oncologists?" *The Oncology Journal* 29, no. 10 (October 2015).

Tauber, Alfred I. 2005. *Patient Autonomy and the Ethics of Responsibility*. Cambridge: MIT Press.

Temel, Jennifer S. et al. "Early Palliative Care for Patients with Metastatic Non-Small-Cell Lung Cancer." *New England Journal of Medicine* 363, no. 8 (August 19, 2010).

Thomas, Katie. "In Race for Medicare Dollars, Nursing Home Care May Lag." *New York Times* (April 14, 2015).

Truog, Robert D. "Medical Futility." *Georgia State University Law Review* (2009).

Tucker, Kathryn. Accessed TK, http://www.drlc@lls.edu.

Turse, Nick. "For America, Life Was Cheap in Vietnam." *The New York Times* (October 9, 2013). http://www.nytimes.com/2013/10/10/opinion/for-america-life-was-cheap-in-vietnam.html.

University of California at Berkeley. http://www.demog.berkeley.edu/~andrew/1918/figure2.html.

University of Pennsylvania. "US Settles Case of Gene Therapy Study that Ended with Teen's Death." *University of Pennsylvania Almanac* 51, no. 21 (February 15, 2015). http://www.upenn.edu/almanac/volumes/v51/n21/gts.html.

Waxman, Daniel A., et al. "The Effect of Malpractice Reform on Emergency Medical Department Care." *New England Journal of Medicine* 371 (October 16, 2014).

Weiss, R. B., et al. "High Dose Chemotherapy for High Risk Primary Breast Cancer: An On-Site Review of the Bezwoda Study." *Lancet* 355, no. 9208 (March 19, 2000): 999–1003.

Welch, H. Gilbert, Lisa Schwartz and Steve Woloshin. 2011. *Overdiagnosed: Making People Sick in the Pursuit of Health*. Boston: Beacon Press.

Whoriskey, Peter. "Doubts about Johns Hopkins Research Have Gone Unanswered, Scientist Says." *Washington Post* (March 11, 2013). https://www.washingtonpost.com/business/economy/doubts-about-johns-hopkins-research-have-gone-unanswered-scientist-says/2013/03/11/52822cba-7c84-11e2-82e8-61a46c2cde3d_story.html.

Wicclair, M. "Autonomy Ethics." *Journal of the American Medical Association* 295, no. 20 (May 24/31, 2006).

Wilson, Duff and David Heath. "The Blood Cancer Experiment: Patients Never Knew the Full Danger of Trials They Staked Their Lives On." *Seattle Times* (2001). http://old.seattletimes.com/uninformed_consent/bloodcancer/story1.html.

Wintrobe, Maxwell M. "The Virtue of Doubt and the Spirit of Inquiry," presidential address to the Association of American Physicians (Atlantic City: May 1965), transcribed by the Association of American Physicians: 78:1. Also quoted in William N. Valentine, "Maxwell Mayer Wintrobe 1901–1986—A Biographical Memoir," National Academy of Sciences (1990).

Wood, Gordon. "The Bleeding Founders." *New York Review of Books* (July 10, 2014).

Wyatt, R., and D. R. Williams. "Racial Bias in Health Care and Health." *Journal of the American Medical Association* 314, no. 6 (August 11, 2015).

Yale Cancer Center and Smilow Cancer Hospital. "Breakthroughs: The Year in Review" (2013): 16. https://medicine,yale.edu/cancer/news/YCC_2013Breakthroughs_020514_177444_12062.pdf.

Yasunaga, Hideo et al. "Collaborative Effects of Bystander-initiated Cardiopulmonary Resuscitation and Prehospital Advanced Cardiac Life Support by Physicians on Survival of Out-of-hospital Cardiac Arrest: A Nationwide Population-based Observational Study." *Critical Care* 14 (November 4, 2010): R199. http://ccforum.com/content/14/6/R199.

Index

About the Author

Aroop Mangalik, MD, retired medical oncologist, attended medical school at King George's Medical College in Lucknow, India, and received specialized training in hematology and oncology at the University of Chicago and the University of Utah. In addition to holding faculty positions at the All India Institute of Medical Sciences, the University of Colorado and the University of New Mexico, he has published 50 papers in peer-reviewed journals, has presented talks and papers at national and international scientific meetings, and has served as principal investigator for numerous research studies.

Along with his patient care, research and teaching activities, he was on the Human Research Review Committee (HRRC) at the University of Colorado and continues in that role at the University of New Mexico. Dr. Mangalik has been instrumental in monitoring and improving ethical research practices at both institutions.

For many years, Dr. Mangalik served as member and chair of the Bioethics Committee of the University of New Mexico. Through his work on the Ethics Committee, as well as in his own practice, which included patients from various cultural backgrounds, among them Native Americans, he has witnessed the social, psychological, and economic impact of illness on patients and families. While he has practiced and taught the common standards of diagnosis and treatments, he has also maintained a questioning attitude toward many medical assumptions. His decisions and recommendations have always been based on the particular assessment of needs for each patient as an individual.

This book is the result of Dr. Mangalik's personal observations and what he learned from patients, families, students, colleagues and scholars over the past five decades.